Happy Father's Day

from

Ralph & Joyce
and Love

Buster Crabbe's
Arthritis Exercise Book

by Buster Crabbe with Raphael Cilento, M.D.

Simon and Schuster 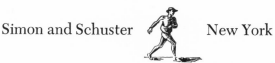 New York

Published by Simon and Schuster
A Division of Gulf & Western Corporation
Simon & Schuster Building
Rockefeller Center
1230 Avenue of the Americas
New York, New York 10020
Designed by Irving Perkins
Manufactured in the United States of America
1 2 3 4 5 6 7 8 9 10

Library of Congress Cataloging in Publication Data

Crabbe, Buster, date.
Buster Crabbe's arthritis exercise book.

Includes index.
1. Arthritics—Rehabilitation. 2. Exercise
therapy. I. Cilento, Raphael, 1931- joint author.
II. Title. III. Title: Arthritis exercise book.
RC933.C75   616.7'2'C624   79-26302

ISBN 0-671-24019-6

Contents

Introduction

Some may find it surprising that I have written a book about arthritis, yet this mysterious affliction has long been a subject of great interest to me. I've seen many friends plagued by this painful disease and its effects can strike almost anyone. Many celebrities, including Katharine Hepburn, Henry Fonda, Joan Fontaine, Betty Ford, James Cagney, Lucille Ball, Jane Wyman and Rock Hudson suffer from arthritis. And as people get older the likelihood of their getting arthritis increases enormously. For a long time my own feeling has been that exercise might help, but not being a medical man I didn't have the training and education to confirm my theories. I had the good fortune to be introduced to Dr. Raphael Cilento, a gifted physician with a special interest in the subject of arthritis. It occurred to us that we might be able to collaborate and produce a book that would combine Dr. Cilento's sound medical approach with my practical experience of exercise and physical fitness through proper diet and weight control.

This book is the result of our teamwork, and I sincerely hope that you find it helpful and informative and that it will bring you or someone you know a measure of freedom from the pain of arthritis.

BUSTER CRABBE

BUSTER CRABBE'S
ARTHRITIS EXERCISE BOOK

CHAPTER ONE

OSTEOARTHRITIS—WHAT IS IT?

More people are crippled by arthritis than by any other disease known to medicine. Three hundred sixty-three million people, which amounts to ten percent of the world's population, have arthritis in one form or another. In our own country, fifty million people have arthritis, and twenty million suffer from it so seriously that they require medical care. This means that arthritis strikes one out of every ten Americans, including twice as many women as men, and at least two hundred fifty thousand children. No one, then, can question the severity of this disease.

In any group of friends over the age of thirty, there are bound to be several, and even a majority, who suffer from this awful malady. And it is common at family reunions or holiday family gatherings for several of the older members, the grandmothers and the grandfathers, to sit in groups and discuss their aches and pains, their backaches and their arthritis. These are not just frivolous complaints. Arthritis is a very serious disease which causes intense pain and immobility, particularly among older people, but also among juveniles and people in their twenties and thirties.

There are over a hundred types of arthritis, and many of these are confused with each other. Arthritis, in general, is the inflammation of the joints. This condition can be caused by many different factors, each one denoting a different type of the general disease, arthritis. Osteoarthritis, the subject of this book, is a degenerative joint disease.

11

Only in the latter part of this century have people begun to probe the causes and to look seriously at ways to treat osteoarthritis and the other crippling forms of arthritis. Unfortunately, the surface has just been scratched, and countless people are still suffering from the grave deformities brought on by the disease. For example, the son of an old friend of mine, who as a child was a very promising violinist, became afflicted with osteoarthritis just at the beginning of his professional career. For several months we all hoped that the disease would remit so that Jonathan could continue his musical career. However, to his grief and the anguish of his friends and family, the joints of his hands became so inflamed and so painful, that Jonathan could no longer even move the bow across the strings of the violin. He was forced to give up his music completely.

Norma, a childhood friend of my wife's, worked all her life as a dancing teacher for small children. Not only had she spent a long and fulfilling life at her dance studio, but she also loved to cook big family dinners for her own three children and seven grandchildren. She also spent hours on weekends and during summer vacations teaching her granddaughters how to sew and crochet.

Norma was truly an example to us of how to find the greatest pleasure in the simple things in life. She and her husband, an insurance executive, looked forward to spending a pleasurable retirement in a mobile home park near Palm Springs in southern California. At this park many recreational facilities were offered, such as tennis, golf, swimming, bridge, and horseback riding. After only three months of this wonderful and much-deserved life, Norma was diagnosed as having osteoarthritis. She could no longer participate in the sports, for her arms and knees were beginning to stiffen up, and they gave her much pain. The doctors did everything they could to ease the aching in her joints with drugs, but no medicine could completely relieve it, nor could any drug take away the stiffness. After two years, Norma was even forced to quit playing bridge at the park's clubhouse-lounge: she could not even hold the cards without experiencing pain.

Until recently these people, and countless others, have been offered little or no relief from their miseries. We know that nutrition, exercise, and emotions affect the body more than any other factors, and we know that in healing any disease, we must pay attention to these.

I have spent most of my life learning how to maintain health through proper exercise. Now, my old friends come to me and ask me for advice about pain they suffer because of arthritis. I have found that most doctors are too busy treating fatal diseases to have time to concern themselves with making the arthritic patient more comfortable. Consequently, millions of people feel that they must put up with the pain, that there is no real comfort in sight for them. This results in people becoming less active—they simply cannot move or participate in certain activities for the pain they would experience. Of course, this forms a vicious circle. Inactive people with arthritis will grow stiffer, not only because of the arthritis, but also because of the inactivity, which in turn, will produce more pain.

When my friends came to me for advice, I at first could only tell them that I knew the vicious circle had to be cracked somehow. Today I have seen that certain kinds of exercise, if done faithfully, not only relieve the pain of arthritis, but also break through this vicious circle, allowing people to lead happy, healthy, and normal lives.

A DEFINITION OF OSTEOARTHRITIS

Osteoarthritis is one of the more severe forms of arthritis. It claims approximately ten million sufferers in the United States. It, like most types of arthritis, is a painful joint disease, but the pain and inflammation occur because of wear and tear on the joints. The condition comes about, then, because of aging of the joints. Those joints that carry the most body weight are subjected to the greatest stress, and consequently the spine, the knees, and the hips are the ones affected. The wrists, the elbows, the shoulders, and the ends of the fingers can also be affected.

Osteoarthritis is commonly thought to be an old man's disease, but this opinion lately has been shown to be a fallacy. Patients develop osteoarthritis as early as age twenty or thirty, as has been shown by histological evidence and X rays. However, the aching, stiffness, and creaking of the joints do not appear until middle age. Osteoarthritis is not a systemic disease. It does not affect the entire body. It attacks joints locally. Although an older person, or a younger person with weak joints, can experience a deterioration of many joints all over the body at the same time, each of these joints is a separate problem. Osteoarthritis attacks these joints in isolation from each other, and the problem goes on for years. Seldom is it seen to remit.

The most common joint to be attacked, with the most serious consequences, is the hip joint. Thousands of people with this type of arthritis have experienced permanent crippling of their hips. Some amount of hip replacement has been made possible, but for the most part, people with arthritis of the hips suffer an increasing deformity of the joint and eventually lose their ability to walk. One woman, a world-famous ice skater in the 1930s, began to suffer from stiffening around her thigh and waist. She ignored the difficulty for many months, performing complicated turns and stunts all the while. Eventually, she started feeling pain while performing. In the course of the year, the pain localized to her hip and she was diagnosed as having arthritis in that joint. She continued skating for several years, trying all kinds of cures such as warm wax, heat treatments, salt immersions, and copper bands, finally relying on drugs to kill the pain. Ultimately she was forced to quit professional skating. A terribly courageous woman, she remained as active as possible all her life, teaching and choreographing skate numbers for ice spectacles and motion pictures, but she was unable to continue with her first love of performing. There are thousands of other people who have been afflicted with this kind of hip arthritis, particularly crippling because it presents such an obstacle to normal, functional activities such as walking.

Osteoarthritis, then, is caused by the aging of the joints. It would be comforting to believe that we are the same people throughout all our lives. We, of course, can be healthy people always, but as we grow older, inescapable changes in our bodies occur, affecting the level of health. Changes occur in the joints, bones, muscles, and tendons. Most of these changes are painless. We wake up one morning and notice a few gray hairs silvering into the blond or black, or we look in the mirror at night and see tiny crinkles around our eyes. These are parts of the normal process of aging. Unfortunately, other parts of the body are not as painless when they grow old. When joints deteriorate they become painful and inflamed, and it is more than a psychological problem that the individual must deal with.

To understand what happens when joints deteriorate to cause arthritis, we must first understand how a joint works. There is a space that is filled with lubricating fluid. Any joint, be it mechanical or one in the human body, needs lubrication in order to function. When you take your car in for a lube job, you are asking the mechanic to grease the joints so there will be less friction when the car operates. The lubrication system of the joints in a human body works in much the same way. The two surfaces where the bones meet, the cartilage coating, have a high natural slipperiness. They are somewhat like certain kinds of plastic that are self-lubricating. When we walk or sit or move in any way, our bones move against each other, thus utilizing our joints. When pressure is applied to a joint, that is to say, when we move our bodies at all, the self-lubricating aspect of this cartilage coating over the bones at our joints becomes especially important, for extra lubrication is produced just where it is needed. In other words, when the bones press against each other, the fluid between them thickens so as to create a smoother movement of the body. If for some reason the lubrication-producing cartilage is damaged, the resulting breakdown ultimately causes inflammation and pain in the joints, which is the beginning of arthritis.

There are three major reasons why joints will become damaged. The first is that we grow older and our joints wear out. The second reason is that each time our joints rub together an infinitesimal amount of abrasion occurs and eventually this scars the surface, the cartilage, so that the fluid can no longer be secreted. The third reason is that the breakdown occurs due to repeated impact shock. This reason relates as much to the bones as to the lubricating cartilage surface. The bones in the body have a certain elasticity. In jumping and running they absorb some of the force of the impact, but when our bones stiffen, as they do when we grow older, they become less elastic and the impact shock on the cartilage is harder. Other reasons for occurrence of osteoarthritis include joints that do not fit together as they should—in other words, joints that are malformed, even slightly, from birth or as a result of accidents—and chemical or biological changes that occur in the body, causing joint breakdown, too.

These are reasons why joints become damaged. The development of this process, or the worsening of an osteoarthritic condition, takes a fairly long time to occur. The first changes in the structure of the joints are usually infinitesimal, and they occur in childhood. These changes do not, as a rule, cause any pain at this point. By the time a person reaches his or her twenties or thirties the changes have developed to the point where they can be seen under an X ray. The pain and deformity, though, don't start until the person has reached his forties or fifties. At this point the condition is an annoyance as opposed to a serious disease. We may feel slight aches around our joints from time to time, but no severe pain. The joints, though, like the entire body, respond to the new level of development by making an attempt to heal themselves. To counteract the now deformed cartilage at the edges of the joints, new cartilage grows over it and forms a hard knob which later becomes bony. Unfortunately, these bony, knobby irregularities at the joints serve to aggravate the problem, and by the time the person reaches old age intense pain and deformity have usually become a part of daily life.

WHO GETS ARTHRITIS?

Sixty percent of the population over age sixty experience some form of osteoarthritis. This does not mean that it is an older person's disease solely, or that everyone afflicted is totally immobilized. Thousands and thousands of people suffer milder forms which may or may not start as early as childhood. As we have seen, whenever the lubricating cartilage becomes deformed, the joints begin to malfunction and to cause pain and inflammation. This may happen at any time during a person's life, and to any degree of severity.

I know of many executives who have begun to suffer from mild forms of osteoarthritis, and who are able to continue working. One in particular, the vice president in charge of advertising at a large weekly newspaper in Arizona, has in the last three years gotten arthritis in his elbows and knees.

He still goes to work every day, and while his activities have been modified somewhat, his secretary taking on much of the actual physical work, his job is such that he hasn't had to stop working. He was lucky he was not an outdoor worker, but the condition he was in when we spoke the first time, before he started practicing these exercises, was still one of great discomfort.

We met at a party on a hot evening in Arizona. He was standing on the patio, which immediately made me curious, because all the people at the party were either swimming in the pool or lying on chaise longues on the patio next to the pool. I walked over and began talking to him, and he told me that his knees were hurting too much for him to sit down, that he felt better standing up. He explained that he had developed mild aches in his joints two years before, and that he had tried all sorts of remedies, from drugs which the doctor did not want to give him too often because the pain was not terribly great, to warm baths which relieved the ache only for short periods, to copper bracelets which did not help at all. He told me that he had finally learned to live with the ache, as you might a toothache. Although I thought it admirable that he could teach himself to cope with the pain, I did not envy his life of a "constant toothache." Here was a man, then, whose practical life was only slightly affected, yet I am sure the psychological effects of enduring this persistent pain could only have been detrimental. Think of the mood you are in when you have a toothache, how you are irritable and snap at your friends and family and generally want to be left alone. Now, if you knew that the condition would continue all of your life and that you would always be in that mood, think of how the irritation would multiply. So this condition, too, seems to be intolerable, though in a very different way from the condition of people who are crippled.

There is no particular set of people who get arthritis. It hits every segment and every occupation, from executives to

housewives to athletes to electricians. While the greater inci-
dence of this disease occurs as people grow older, it is certainly not limited to senior citizens. Teenagers and young
people in their twenties have been known to become afflicted
with it, also.

CHAPTER TWO

CATCH IT EARLY— TREAT IT RIGHT

Oftentimes, as we have seen, osteoarthritis begins early in life, in the mid-thirties, say, as just an annoying ache that we learn to live with. Like the advertising executive in Arizona, many people experience mild pains around their joints and simply refuse to admit that anything serious might be occurring. Until the pain becomes intense, it is assumed by the suffering individual to be unimportant.

A friend of mine in Los Angeles said to me one day, "Sure, I have these aches in my elbows. But look, if it is arthritis, what can they do? The doctor'll give me a lot of aspirin or shoot me up with pain killers and maybe the pain will stop for a while, but I can't go around all day all filled up with dope. I've got to go to work. I've got to support my family. I'd just as soon ignore the whole thing. If it gets worse, then I'll go. Besides, everyone knows they can't cure it. What's the use of going to a doctor for something they can't help?"

This is an understandable and common attitude. However, it is just the sort of attitude that foments situations where people end up by experiencing incredible levels of pain. It is essential to get treatment for arthritis early. To ignore going to the doctor is to live in ignorance as to the extent and the exact nature of your condition. Also, with the new interest that medical science is developing in all forms of arthritis today, it is doubly essential to go for diagnosis early, for many new methods of treatment of this painful disease are opening up.

TREATMENTS OF THE PAST

Once a person with osteoarthritis has decided to go to a doctor, what kind of outlook will he find there? We must remember that arthritis has always been thought of as being a "chronic" disease. What this means is that it cannot be cured, and that the condition will accelerate throughout the person's life. Consequently, *until today*, the picture of the future of an osteoarthritic has been, indeed, a discouraging one.

For decades doctors have prescribed all manner of remedies to comfort the patient, to cover or temporarily relieve the pain. Few doctors have had the time to seriously consider the plight of the discouraged arthritic who must constantly be taking or trying drugs and treatments without any hope of permanently alleviating his condition. A person who goes to a doctor and is told that there is no cure for his condition, and that the only thing he can do is to take massive doses of aspirin to kill the pain, will turn out to be a very disheartened individual. Unfortunately, time and time again this is exactly what happens. People are sent home with directions to take anywhere between twenty and thirty aspirins a day to relieve their pain. Besides being only a temporary measure, these large amounts of aspirin serve to burn out the patient's stomach, thus causing other forms of illness. No wonder osteoarthritics become resigned and end up simply learning to cope with the pain.

A wealth of these "camouflage" treatments has been offered in the past. Aside from mere aspirin, there is a whole range of pain-reducing and pain-killing drugs. Unfortunately it is the case that the milder drugs do little good and the stronger ones, while easing the pain, wreak havoc on the patient's body in other ways. One friend of mine could barely walk from the deformity and pain in her knee joints. Her doctor tried several other treatments and drugs, and ultimately decided to give her cortisone. Susanna took the shots for several months, and the pain subsided; but as a result of the cortisone, her face and stomach bloated out to unnatural proportions, and the blood vessels in her arms began to break down. They would break just beneath the skin, giving her a horrid-looking latticework of purple veins all across her arms. She was forced to quit taking the cortisone, and until she began the schedule of exercises, she was again in constant pain.

There are treatments outside of the drug range, too. Oftentimes doctors will prescribe and apply hot wax to the inflamed area, which acts as a form of warming insulation. Ice packs, to reduce swelling and inflammation and also to numb the pain, have been used. Recently a few doctors have introduced acupuncture into the list of possible treatments.

Hip surgery, also a relatively new form of treatment, is being used more and more. Arthritis of the hip is, of course, one of the most crippling kinds. Earlier forms of surgery, while they might have relieved pain, always left the patient with an awkward, unsightly limp. Of late, however, a great revolution in modern treatment of this disease has come about with the name of hip replacement arthroplasty. This surgery was developed by British doctors. It involves replacing human hip joints, or the bone, with artificial metal or plastic joints. These are glued into the patient's own bones with a special cement developed solely for surgical purposes. When the operation is successful, the patient enjoys a nearly normal life with a hip that gives no pain and functions as well as a natural hip. A hip of this sort lasts for fifteen years or more before it needs to be replaced. For older and more frail patients, the strain on the hip tends to be less, and the life span of the artificial joint will be longer than that of its owner. This form of surgery can be performed on nearly everyone, regardless of age. It has been known to be successful on patients over ninety who would otherwise be confined to their beds as helpless cripples. Patients are up and walking after such surgery within two to three weeks. The modern form of this kind of surgery has only been used for about seven years. The unfortunate aspect of it is that it is radical surgery, and quite expensive. Many times just the people who would benefit from it most, the elderly living on social security or tight pension budgets, cannot afford this type of surgery.

There are also several forms of earlier treatment which were out-and-out quackery, whether intentional or misguided, or which were simply fads, however scientific. All of these need to be mentioned here. For several years it has been the practice to prescribe large doses of Vitamin D and cod liver oil for arthritic patients. The purpose of this was to alter the balance of calcium and phosphorus in the body, yet it has never been found that these elements have a known causative effect on an arthritic condition. Along these lines, Vitamin C has also been prescribed in large doses, also on the basis of insufficient evidence or misinformed opinions.

Exposure to radioactivity was a very popular treatment in certain western states. People were taken into abandoned uranium mines and were exposed to small amounts of radioactivity. For one reason or another there were several of these people whose conditions began to improve, and this was immediately and mythically attributed to the radioactivity treatments. While this kind of exposure probably did no physical harm, it also did absolutely no good. There is no scientific basis for this treatment.

Vaccines of many types have also been used to treat

arthritis, but these have no beneficial effect on deformed arthritic joints either.

Injection of sulfur is another type of treatment that was used in the middle of this century. However, there has never been discovered a particular sulfuric imbalance in the bodies of arthritic patients, so injection of sulfur into the body would not be of any use because it would not be correcting anything. Immersion in warm sulfur baths, on the other hand, has long been claimed to have curative effects. The essential element here, though, is the heat of the water. The pain in the joints is eased because the water is warm and it buoys up the body. The same effect can be achieved at home, in the bathtub, as opposed to an expensive health spa. Unfortunately, this treatment is only a temporary one, and as soon as the body temperature drops, the pain in the joints recurs.

A peculiar treatment became popular in the last sixty years. This is the use of certain kinds of venom for treatment of arthritis. The two major kinds of venom employed are bee venom and cobra venom. Bee venom became popular because it was claimed that bee keepers are not known to suffer from arthritis. This is a totally unsubstantiated belief, and results from injection of bee venom have been not only ineffective, but they have been found at times to be harmful. Cobra and other snake venoms were also used, but again there was no scientific support for this treatment.

Another treatment, spinal pumping, was developed by an Austrian doctor in 1939, who claimed that arthritis was an abnormality of the nervous system. Consequently, he injected spinal fluid into his patients, and claimed excellent results. However, doctors have not been able to reproduce these results, and the treatment is generally a dangerous one.

Several serums and other drugs have from time to time been used, such as antireticular cytotoxic serum, chaulmoogra oil (a one-time treatment of leprosy), penicillin, sulfa drugs, iodides, and arsenic. None of these has ever been proven to have recurring, consistent, satisfying success. Many times the clear hope of the patient in trying "one last treatment" is the most beneficial part of the remedy.

An extremely popular yet irrational treatment for arthritis which had a tidal wave of commercialism throughout the country a few years ago was chlorophyll. This element was turned into a product by several Madison Avenue scoundrels, and was manufactured for everything from fertilizers to toothpaste to fly paper, and of course, inevitably, to a remedy for arthritis. It was touted as being "nature's own cure," and publicized for the fact that chlorophyll was the basis of all life and contained the healing rays of the sun. Of course, the logic here fails miserably. Simply because chlorophyll is involved in plant life processes does not mean that human beings can benefit from it. And it certainly does not mean that the particular disease of arthritis will be cured by it. Indeed, the human body is far too complex to be able to be cured according to these simplistic, ill-thought-out remedies.

And aside from this wide range of quack-like, pseudo-scientific treatments, there is, of course, the realm of mystical, superstitious "treatments" which simply serves to perpetuate the myths of arthritis. These are charms and amulets. For centuries copper has been said to be a cure for arthritis. Even today, people still wear copper plates in their shoes or copper wrist bands to alleviate their pain. If, by chance, the pain does slacken certain days, this cannot be attributed to the copper. Nor can the wearing of blue glass beads from Turkey be said to keep more serious illness from an arthritic. I knew one poor woman who had been bounced from so many different treatments to others that she finally bought several glass beads from a Turkish "gypsy" and put them in each room of her house. When I asked her about the effectiveness of this "remedy" she told me that in fact it was quite scientific. She said that the glass beads absorbed certain elements in the air which normally caused moisture to get into her bones and that with the presence of these beads, her body was allowed to remain normal. How sorry I felt for this woman, yet how silly the whole theory seemed to me. In no way could the beads have helped, but her desperation was such that she would have done anything, would have believed anything.

The list of supposed treatments is endless. Alfalfa tea and fever therapy and special garters and oscilloclast detectors and various quack chiropractics. They are too numerous to go into in any detail. What remains when the smoke of the failure of all of these methods clears, is that none can cure permanently, and even the best are only temporary camouflages of the pain.

CONTEMPORARY LIFESTYLES

I have learned in all my years of healthful activity and of dealing with all aspects of keeping the body in shape, that at the core of the healthy life are two elements: proper diet and proper exercise. These elements not only affect the totality of a person's life, but they *create* that life. A person who does not eat properly, who consumes much alcohol and sugar and greasy foods and starches, can never be free from illnesses. Likewise, a person who sits in an office all day, or a woman who chain-smokes in the shade of a darkened living room after cleaning the kitchen in the morning, will always suffer from ailments, and will be more prone to be a sufferer from arthritis than a more agile, well-nourished person.

These are simple facts that any doctor will tell you. Yet our society, even in light of these facts, does not take them into account. Our society sets up situations where a person's daily life consists of a quick toast and coffee breakfast, often with some jam on the toast to add a bit of flavor and to take the place of the real flavor of a hearty meal. Very often, too, there's the quick instant sugary orange juice which is frequently not orange juice but only a synthetic concoction, shot up with artificial Vitamin C and sweetened to taste good. A person who starts the day in this way cannot hope to have an energetic, satisfying day.

Which is just as well. Because this same person, be he executive or secretary, will rush off to work and spend the entire morning in a cloistered office. In a chair. Tense and having no real way to alleviate the tension.

The next step in the working day is, of course, to eat a huge, unhealthy, greasy lunch at a restaurant with people from the office; after which the individual goes back to sitting for the rest of the day.

At five o'clock he or she goes home, too exhausted mentally and physically from the lack of real nutrition to perform any exercise. So the person waits, reads or watches television until dinner, and then eats perhaps the only healthy meal of the day. But to eat a "balanced" meal this late in the day is useless. The energy gained by this meal is wasted, as the person usually simply sits around the house until bedtime. The "energy" then turns to fat, for it is not needed in the metabolism.

Is it no wonder that we are a society of unhealthy people, susceptible to any and every kind of disease and virus? Specifically in terms of arthritis, we are unused to any kind of exercise, so naturally our joints will stiffen up early; once stiff, we will not want to exercise or move them, because after all, we did not even get proper exercise when we were young.

In terms of diet, most people carry from ten to twenty-five pounds of excess weight, which is extremely harmful to an arthritic for the already strained joints feel even more strain the more weight they have to carry and shift. Consequently, our lifestyle is set up to intensify an arthritic condition. This is the vicious circle I spoke of earlier. The stiffer a person's joints get, the more he will not want to move, yet the more he does not move, the more pain and stiffness there will be. I am not by any means suggesting a strenuous game of tennis for a man of sixty who has been afflicted with arthritis. The exercise must be slow in beginning, increasing in gradual increments, and the program must be quite controlled. However, I have found that exercise is the healthiest way to relieve joints which are aching from arthritis affliction.

I first began suggesting certain exercises to older friends of mine who were suffering from mild arthritic pain. One by one they began coming back to me and asking for more exercises, or for variations, or for "permission" to continue the original ones only more strenuously. We found, on a pretty much hit-and-miss basis, that the exercises began to improve the conditions of these people. Not all at once, mind you. This is not to say—like the exponents of so many "fad" plans—that my exercises will immediately cure arthritis and eliminate any pain. That would be a frivolous and totally untrue assertion. If anyone ever claims such a thing, and many people do, you can be assured that it is a false claim. To this day there is no known absolute cure for arthritis. However, a solid program of de-stiffening exercises can indeed relieve much of the pain. As with several of my friends who have been practicing these exercises for a number of years now, even most of the pain can be eliminated.

Success in these exercises depends on the enthusiasm and thoroughness with which the patient and his family approach them.

This is very much a "do it yourself" program. From my suggestions, you can proceed to work out a plan of activity which will best suit your own day and your own occupation. *Naturally, it is important to consult and to use the guidance of your private physician* in any and all health-oriented programs you adopt.

Also, it is important to realize, in the light of present knowledge of the disease, that any treatment is a lifelong treatment.

It is unwise to begin a program with the idea that in a few weeks or a few months, after your joints have ceased aching, you will go back to your previous pattern of life. For just as arthritis is a lifelong malady, the alleviation of pain from arthritis must likewise last your whole life. Fortunately, I have been told time and time again that not only do my exercises help modify and at times eliminate the pain, but they also forge happier, healthier lives for those who use them. This of course is the case with any exercise program. It is natural for the body to be exercised, for all parts of the body to be utilized, to be toned. When muscles are sluggish, this is an unnatural state. People need to move about. Our bodies are basically resilient, self-healing mechanisms. It is only when we let them get out of condition that the self-healing and the resiliency disappear. So it is only natural that this program of exercises would not only ease the pain of arthritis, but would improve the overall health of each practitioner.

I have never had a person fail to improve his health while following my plan, just as I have never had one who did not notice substantial lessening of pain after the first two to three weeks. Along the same lines, people are very encouraged by the new feelings of energy, and the loss of pain and stiffness; I have never known one person who followed my plan and who felt the improvement, stop doing these exercises. There have been those who quit early on, but none who have continued long enough to see the results have ever thrown in the towel. They are all happier, healthier, pain-free people today.

Steve, a fourteen-year-old boy, came to my home one afternoon. Despite his shyness, I could tell that he was quite determined about getting some straight answers and opinions from me. He explained that he wanted to be a doctor some day, and already knew about several illnesses, one of which was arthritis, and he was convinced that he had the beginnings of it in his wrist. He had complained to his parents about this, but they, of course, assumed that it was only a future medical student's hypochondria.

After speaking with him for several hours, I realized that he was wiser than his years. Consequently I took him to a next-door neighbor who was a doctor. After a quick examination, the doctor suspected that indeed it was arthritis. We subsequently phoned Steve's parents and arranged for a thorough examination. After this, it was confirmed to be arthritis in the wrist in the earliest stages. The doctor prescribed various mild medications. However, being a neighbor, he knew of my arthritis exercise program, and he asked me to work with Steve on developing such a program for him. I did this, and Steve, being a conscientious and thorough boy, followed them carefully. This sort of program was almost second nature to him. Today, Steve has no trace of arthritic problems, no pain, and no deformity. He has just graduated from medical school and will be interning in New York City at a major hospital which has a fine clinic specializing in arthritis. We have stayed in close contact, and will continue to remain so. I am quite proud of him.

In contrast to Steve's eagerness is the story of another friend of mine, a draftsman named Will. I first met him at Marina del Rey in Los Angeles. He kept his sailboat there and we used to chat across the bows quite frequently. The most noticeable thing about Will was his broad smile as he puttered about his sailboat. Every weekend I would see him out there, painting and polishing and scraping down the hull. Over the years I learned to know him as a very friendly, yet quite stubborn and independent man. He was the epitome of the West Coast man. One summer he stopped frequenting the marina, and appeared only about once a month. When I asked him why, he replied that his "old bones were aching." He would always laugh after he said this, but I knew there must have been much truth in it for him to forgo one of the greatest joys in his life. As it turned out, Will had had arthritis all along, and had ignored it all the years I knew him, until finally it flared up to such an extent that he could not stand the pain.

His doctor prescribed several varieties of pain-killers. Will took them faithfully for several months, but he finally realized that although the problem was suppressed, it was not alleviated. Even though he was relatively pain-free while under the effects of the drugs, he still could not putter around the sailboat as before, because of stiffness and discomfort which a pain-killer could never remove. Being the independent man that he was, he resented having constantly to ingest or be shot up with foreign substances. Will had simply lost his zest for life.

One day he and his wife came down to the boat for a quiet picnic. It was then that I casually bet him that he would see improvement in his condition if he would try my exercises. Will was not the type to take this sort of advice, even from a close friend, but he was also not the type to pass up a bet, even from a stranger. He began exercising that very day, doing some mild forms of twists and stretches. Within a few short weeks his condition was radically improved. He no longer needed the pain-killers, and the stiffness had abated somewhat. After three months of exercising, he was back on the boat each weekend, puttering around as the old Will I used to know. However, Will has learned the hard way that it is essential to continue exercising, because the moment he stops, the pain returns.

Trina, the thirty-year-old secretary at the television studio in Hollywood where I used to film one of my TV shows, developed arthritis in her upper back. At that time she was quite overweight and physically very unfit. We used to joke about making gym dates where she might get some proper exercise, but none of these suggestions ever got beyond the joke stage. As it was, Trina could not even walk up a flight of stairs without getting out of breath and needing to rest.

When she first experienced the pains she did not believe that it could be arthritis. Her initial reaction was to climb into bed and phone in sick for several days. Finally, she returned to work, but the pains remained. She went to the studio doctor and was diagnosed as having arthritis. They immediately put her on a mild pain-killer and gave her heat treatments. I tried to talk her into exercising a little to relieve some of the stiffness in her back. Although it was completely against Trina's nature, the pain was intense enough and the exercises were easy enough, so that she began the program.

After a few weeks she found the pain diminishing. Not only that, but for the first time in her life, she was carrying out a healthful plan of regular exercise. She found that this plan was enjoyable, and it helped her lose weight and tone up her muscles. At her young age, she had a full life to look forward to. It is fortunate that the arthritis has gone into remission and, just as important, that she has learned a healthier, more vital way of life. Those old jokes about dates at the gym are no longer jokes. It is every afternoon that you can find Trina working out on her lunch break at the studio gym, which she follows with a quick swim in the pool. Trina has become a vibrant, lovely and healthy young woman.

One of the most surprising occurrences of arthritis I have seen was in my family doctor, Lou. I was in his office one day for my routine check-up when I noticed that the joints of his fingers were swollen into shiny-skinned knobs. I asked him what had happened to his hands. He replied that recently his arthritis had worsened, and the joints of his fingers and wrists had swollen up. He also mentioned that if it weren't for the drugs he was taking, he would be in considerable pain. Although he was a doctor, this did not help him much in treating his own condition effectively. Again, drugs were no answer and there was no cure in sight for his malady.

Naturally, I was a little hesitant to suggest my program, regardless of how effective I had found it to be. After all, Lou was the doctor! Besides, I had discussed it with him occasionally before, when I first began to develop the theory. He didn't seem too eager at this point to discuss it, not even enough to ask me about it. But I trusted my own judgment, and I casually suggested that he exercise his hands to alleviate the stiffness caused by the arthritis in the inflamed joints. Lou was quite skeptical about this. Being a doctor, he was well aware of all the latest scientific treatments of arthritis, but he had not read any journal articles on the subject of exercise as treatment for arthritis. Exercise seemed far too simple a solution for this long-incurable disease. When I saw his skeptical frown, I asked him, quite abruptly, to make a fist with his hand. He could not. Yet after he tried, and tried again, the fingers would close a little farther than before. This, I told him, was the principle behind my program of treatment.

He decided that he had nothing to lose in trying my suggestions. He began with several fist-clenching and finger-separation exercises, and he continued these for several weeks faithfully. Soon the pain began to diminish and the swelling went down. In a couple of months he was back to performing all of the office tasks that a doctor should do, but that lately he had turned over to his nurse. He now continues the exercises, and also prescribes similar programs for his own patients who become afflicted with arthritis.

As we have seen, it is important to recognize the seriousness of this disease, and to go for treatment early in its development. To wait is only to remain in ignorance and to prolong the pain. The most effective form of treatment that I have ever seen is that of a faithful, sensible program of exercises which you can develop for yourself (and of course under the supervision of your doctor), and which you can carry out at home.

The next chapters will deal with the basics and the directions for this program of exercises.

CHAPTER THREE

INDOOR EXERCISES— THE BASIC PLAN

Generally, we can think of joints as one would think of shocks on a car. The bouncier the ride, the more stress that is put on the shock absorbers. With time, shock absorbers wear out and must be replaced. Unfortunately, in the human body when joints begin to wear out they cannot be replaced. Consequently they begin to ache, to swell, to become inflamed, and to stiffen: all indications of degeneration of the joints. So, to counteract this condition, the answer is *not* to remain, or to become *more*, inactive, as many medical people would have you believe. This only aggravates the stiffness. Rather, the answer is to slowly loosen the stiffness, restore the elasticity, and thus reduce the pain. This means that we must carefully screen all exercises. Exercises must be of a particular type only. Obviously, exercises that joggle and bounce the bones and body about will be destructive exercises, because they put unneeded strain on the joints and require more cushioning fluid to be secreted from the cartilaginous surfaces at the joints.

However, stretches and elongating exercises are extremely beneficial. It is vital to avoid short, choppy and violent exercises. In general, we must practice large and sweeping movements. A set of circular calisthenics for the arms is advised. Rotating movements for the shoulders and neck are good, but these must never be choppy, too quick, or too violent. In regard to the spine, it is important to practice mild back and side bends which stretch your body the length of the spine, in addition to steady turning or twisting at the waist and rotating the body from side to side. For the legs, stretches and deep knee bends are ideal. And of course, walking, and supine exercises with your legs in the air, are terrific ways to loosen arthritic stiffness.

These stretching exercises, when combined with a balanced diet as prescribed by your doctor plus adequate rest each day (which also means not *too much* rest) form my program of relief from osteoarthritis.

It is essential to begin the program quite slowly. It is always advisable to exercise after a hot bath, when your joints are more supple and less tender than usual. After several weeks, and of course for outdoor and office exercises, it is not necessary always to have a hot bath first. However in the beginning it is essential.

The first day, choose a time at which your mind is free of major worries, *i.e.*, don't begin immediately after coming home from work or after cleaning the house. The mornings are good for many people. It is a good idea always to exercise at the same time of day. This will set up a routine for you, and so on days when you are not inclined to jump right into your schedule of exercises, the momentum of your routine will carry you along. Take a hot bath, not so hot that it will make you lethargic, but warm enough to loosen up your joints and ease the ache a bit. After the bath, relax a few minutes, to bring your body temperature back to normal, and then begin your exercises. The first day you will only work out for about fifteen minutes. This will increase by one exercise (two to three minutes) each day until you have reached a program which lasts for thirty minutes.

After you have done the exercises for one week, consistently, you should begin to notice bodily changes. You should feel more relaxed, notice a diminishing of pain, and of course the stiffness should be lessening. Another way to measure improvement is to take a tape measure, or to have a friend do it for you, and measure the circumference of the joint above and below the main joint-place. This will give you an idea of the increasing muscle bulk, which in turn, indicates newly acquired muscle strength.

It is important to begin each session with a clear feeling in your body. Stand in the middle of your exercise space, as straight as you can, and breathe deeply several times, relaxing after each exhalation. Straighten your body and relax it three times. Hold your arms out to the sides of the room, palms up, and lean your head back, so as to look at the ceiling. Do this gently, and do not strain yourself. If any pain occurs, you are leaning too far. These are not corrective exercises yet; this portion of the program is merely a clearing "wake up" practice. You should begin each session with one to two minutes of this, and end each session in the same way.

The first week, choose three exercises and perform two or three repetitions of each. The repetitions will be increased by two each week until you reach ten to twelve repetitions of a set of approximately ten exercises. This is prescribed for the first two to three months of your recovery. In later chapters I will discuss added strength and maintenance exercises. It is important to remember that in the course of the beginning program, a little strain is desirable. To do a series of exercises and feel nothing, not even the smallest amount of discomfort, is usually a sign that you are doing them incorrectly. However, if you begin to feel actual, intense pain, or if you feel pain after performing the exercises, you are doing them too strenuously and should modify your program.

THE EXERCISES

There are four basic kinds of exercises:

1. *Passive exercise.* This is exercise done by having some-one else move a part of your body. In this case the patient does nothing but relax. Quite often this sort of exercise precedes active movement, or is used when a certain amount of de-stiffening is required. This prevents, then, shortening of muscles, and is most commonly beneficial for people who are bedridden.
2. *Muscle setting.* This is accomplished by the individual's contracting his muscles, holding them a few seconds, then releasing them. This is useful when a joint is so swollen or painful that it is not manipulable. In using these exercises, the muscles around the joint can be moved and worked with, without actually moving the painful joint.
3. *Active exercise.* This is exercise which the patient does himself. This comprises the majority of our program, and generally is the most common form of therapeutic exercise.
4. *Resistive exercise.* This is done by having someone else apply force which resists the patient's efforts to move the part. This type is rather like isometrics.

The following is a list and explanation of exercises. You must choose the exercises corresponding to your particular problem. As an example of a program for the first week, a person with elbow osteoarthritis would start with "wake up" exercises (pages 38-41); then do three elbow exercises of his choice, repeating each specific exercise twice (see exercises for the elbow on pages 43-46); and then choose one postural exercise or yoga exercise (see Chapter 4); and finish the session with the "wake up" exercises again.

POSTURAL EXERCISES

These can be done by everyone, regardless of where their arthritis is located. These are general exercises, aimed at eliminating fatigue, muscle spasm, and pains which come from poor posture. Having swollen joints usually means that a person will compensate, will try to relieve the pain by standing or sitting in a different way. This re-shifting of weight usually causes poor posture, and eventually backfires by placing undue strain on parts of the body which were not meant to receive it. Consequently, it is necessary to improve the posture by correcting these bad habits.

1. The Lizard. Lie on your back on a bed or on the floor with your legs straight out before you. Pull tight your buttocks muscles and retract or pull in your stomach muscles until your stomach is flat. While you are doing this, be sure not to hold your breath. Try to get your lower back flat against the bed; this serves to straighten the curve of your lower back. You can also do this exercise lying face down, with a pillow placed under your stomach. This is the basic exercise from which all the other postural ones are built.

2. The Pumping Lizard. Lie on your back with your hands clasped behind your neck. If this is not possible, put them at your sides or wherever is most comfortable. Repeat exercise Number 1. Hold the position and gradually, very slowly, bend one knee. Slide the foot back, and then repeat with the other leg. It is important to hold your back flat and to slide your feet out slowly until your legs are extended completely (Figure 1).

3. The Staring Lizard. Lie on your back, and cross your arms over your chest. Pull in your stomach very slowly, and remember again not to hold your breath. Tighten your buttocks

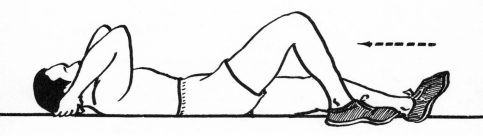

FIGURE 1.

muscles at the same time. Now, slowly and gently raise your head and shoulders from six to eight inches off the bed. Hold for three counts and then lower, again slowly.

4. The Ceiling Reach. Lie on your back again, with your hands at your sides. Pull in your stomach and also tighten your buttocks muscles. Slowly, to a three-count, raise your arms in the air, over your head. While you do this, fill your lungs with air on a three-count inhalation. Now, hold the position for three counts, and then lower your arms and exhale to the same three-count period. While you do this exercise, be sure to keep your back flat against the bed or floor space.

5. The Ground Press. Lie on your back, with your arms at your sides. Pull your buttocks muscles tight and pull your stomach in. Slowly roll your arms outward, and while you do this, turn your palms upward and force your shoulders back. Be sure to press your lower back against the floor or bed. Also, it is important to try to press the back of your neck against the bed, while keeping your chin in.

6. Leg Raises from the Lizard Position. Lie on your back, and if possible place your hands behind your neck. If this is not possible for you, then put them down at your sides. Pull your stomach muscles in, and tuck in your buttocks muscles. With your legs straight, alternately raise and lower first one and then the other. Do this slowly to a count of four on the way up and hold for two, and then four on the way down.

7. *Postural Knee Bends.* Stand with your back against a wall. Your feet should be three inches from the wall, and they should be three inches apart from each other. Put your hands behind your neck. Now, bend your knees as much as possible, also tightening your stomach muscles and tucking in your buttocks muscles. Be sure, while performing this exercise, to keep your back flat against the wall and, after rising, to straighten your knees (Figure 2).

8. *The Swan.* Lie face down on your bed. A pillow should be placed under your stomach. Your arms, shoulders, and

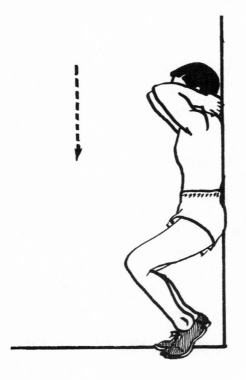

FIGURE 2.

forearms should be extended past the head, but not off the bed, hands touching each other, elbows bent at right angles. Now, tighten your buttocks muscles and pull in your stomach. Slowly, raise your arms and hands from the bed, thus bringing your shoulder blades together. Hold the position for two counts, and then relax slowly, to a count of three (Figure 3).

EXERCISES FOR THE HANDS AND WRISTS

The exercises in this group are aimed at rebuilding hand and finger dexterity and manipulability, and to stop any developing deformity. Our goal is also to reduce pain and increase strength in the hands.

1. Hold your hand relaxed and nearly flat out before you. To a count of four, slowly make a fist, coiling your

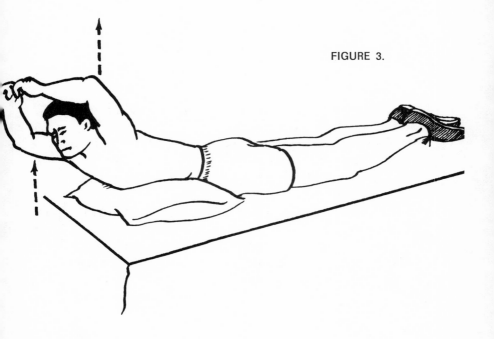

FIGURE 3.

fingers as tight as they will go, short of causing extreme pain. Hold the fist for four counts, and then release slowly, again to a count of four.

2. Stretch your fingers as straight as possible. If, when you do this your fingers are still bent, rest your hand with the palm down on the table. Hold the other hand firmly on top of this hand, and raise the forearm of the hand on the table in an effort to extend the bent fingers (Figure 4).

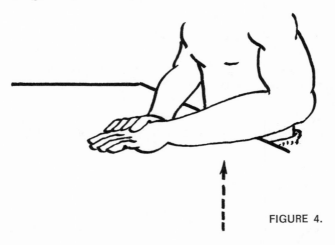

FIGURE 4.

3. Hold your hand out flat in front of you and make an effort to separate the fingers.

4. Touch the end of each finger to the end of the thumb of that same hand; as you do this, make an effort to create as round a circle as possible with the two extended fingers (Figure 5).

5. Hold your hand in front of you and bend it from the wrist as far forward and as far backward as possible. This should be done quite slowly, also, to a count of three. Once flexed, you should hold your hand in the position for three counts, and then bend it forward again.

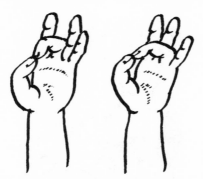

FIGURE 5.

6. Hold your hand before you and slowly and gently move the fingers of the hand toward the thumb of the same hand. When they touch, spring them apart sharply. You should use a four-count as the fingers are moving toward the thumb, but you should move them apart too quickly to register any count.

7. Hold your hand before you, and take the hand with your other hand. Do not squeeze, but hold it gently and turn it back and forth as you might a doorknob. This should be done slowly, but there is no count for it, as you should do it at your own pace.

8. Place your hands on the edge of a table, and with the other hand as opposing force, resist flexing and extending it alternately. This should be done quite slowly, and it is very like isometric exercises.

9. Hold your hands flat together as a person praying might. Slowly, press hands harder and harder against each other, and then relax (Figure 6).

EXERCISES FOR THE ELBOW

The purpose of these exercises is to create enough flexibility in your elbow joint so that you will be able to extend and flex your arms completely. As all sufferers from arthritis are well

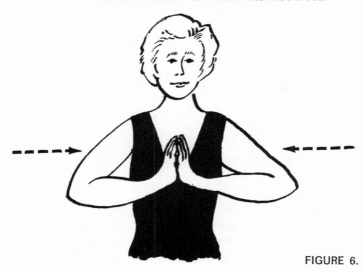

FIGURE 6.

aware, a stiff elbow can keep a person from bringing his hand to his face, and may interfere with such simple but basic tasks as eating, brushing one's hair, shaving, and brushing one's teeth. So an elbow free from pain and stiffness is essential.

1. Lie on your back on the bed, arms along your side. Slowly, with the upper arm resting on the bed, bring the fingers of your hand to the top of your shoulder. Perform this to a count of four, and hold the position for three counts. Then, slowly, relax your arm and bring it back down to the bed so that the entire arm is extended again (Figure 7).

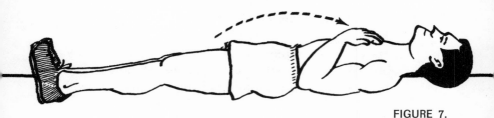

FIGURE 7.

2. Face a wall, approximately twelve inches away. Place your hands, palms flat, upon the surface of the wall. Slowly lean forward, into the wall. Hold the position for three counts, and then resume your previous position (Figure 8).

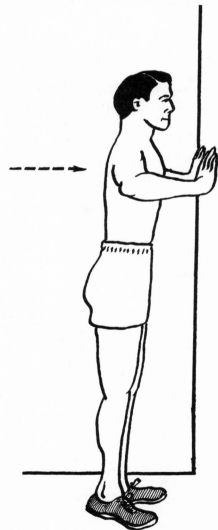

FIGURE 8.

3. Hold one arm straight before you, the elbow straight and rigid as possible. Push with your other hand against the heel of the palm of the rigid hand and arm, while holding that arm still rigid. Do this for three counts and then relax.

EXERCISES FOR THE SHOULDERS AND NECK

The shoulders and neck are essential for most activities. If a person has pain in these areas, chances are that every time he moves he will be in pain. These shoulder exercises combine not only techniques of physical therapy, but they have also been designed by using certain ballet stretches and "carrys," in order to create a proper balance between the various opposing muscles which are at work in any motion made by the shoulders. It is very important to keep the shoulders and neck limber, because inactivity in this area can easily cause adhesions.

1. The Signal Man. Stand in the center of the room, with your arms resting at your sides, the palms of your hands toward your body. Slowly, to a count of three, raise your arm (later alternate with the other one, but only do one arm at a time) sideways as far as possible away from the body. Hold it for two counts and then return it to your side, again to a count of three. Then, also to a count of three, raise it forward, upward, and then as far back as it will go. Hold it for three counts and then return it back down to your side (Figure 9).

2. Supine Arm Carry. Lie on your back with your legs straight and your arms at your sides. Slowly, raise your arm forward and upward as far back as it will go. This should be done to a count of four. Once it is back, swing it slowly

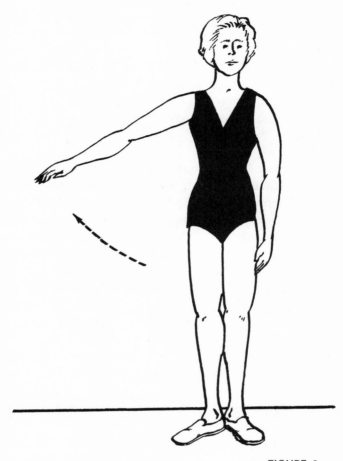

FIGURE 9.

out to the side and back down to the side of your body. This second half of the movement should also be done to a count of four.

3. *Arm Circles.* Stand erect and hold one arm straight out to the side with the elbow unbent. Move the arm in increasingly larger circles, keeping the elbow stiff until the circles brush the side of your leg. Repeat with the other arm.

4. *Stand, Arms Down Alongside Body.* Slowly, and in small circular motions, shrug your shoulders first upward, and then downward until you have completed three circles. These movements make up one exercise, and repetitions should be in threes.

5. *Wall Creep.* There are two parts to this exercise. The first is to stand, facing the wall, with your arm extended directly in front of your body. Touch the wall with your fingertips, and slowly "creep" the fingers up the wall until you have gone as far as you can go. Creep back down again. The second part of the exercise is to stand with your side to the wall; extend your arm again. Touch the wall with your fingers and again creep up the wall and back down.

6. *Stand in the Center of the Exercise Space.* Place your hands at the back of your neck, with your elbows pointed out. Making sure that your elbows continue to point out, bring your hands forward over your head and downward in front of your face and then backward to a count of five to the lower part of the back. Reverse the motion, again to a count of five.

7. *Arm Carry.* Stand with your feet at shoulder width apart. One of your hands should be on a chair for balance. Hold the other arm gently curved before you. Slowly raise it in a graceful arc straight up until it is directly over your head. Follow the movement of it with a slight turn of your head. Continue on back from the high point of the arc, forming a circle in the air, finally letting your arm gradually drop down until it reaches waist level. Bring it around to the original position and repeat. After two repetitions, alternate with your other arm.

EXERCISES FOR THE ANKLES AND TOES

The ankles and toes often are found to be arthritic because all of the weight of the body is centered on them. They take the most strain from being raised up and driven down to the ground constantly. After arthritis has set in and the ankles and toe joints become painful, the person tends always to walk with these joints held rigidly. This of course, makes the joints become stiff, thus accelerating the progress of the arthritis.

1. Foot Flex. Sit on the edge of a table, your feet dangling over the side. Slowly bend one foot up and then down. Repeat using other foot.

2. Still sitting on the bed, turn your foot from left to right very slowly. Relax it while exercising the other one.

3. Foot Rotations. While sitting on the edge of the bed, point your foot out in front of you. Begin to rotate it, making three circles in one direction, and then reversing the motion, making three circles in the other direction. Alternate feet.

4. Sitting on the edge of the bed with your foot and leg extended before you, sling a strap or folded towel under the arch of your foot. Flex your foot from the ankle back toward your body by pulling on the ends of the cloth. Press against this resistance with your foot muscles several times, then relax and repeat with your other foot (Figure 10).

5. Stand against a wall with your back and your heels touching the wall. Your feet should be no more than four inches apart, and preferably less. Gently and carefully slide down the wall, bending your knees and eventually your ankles. Be sure with this exercise to go very slowly, to a count of five,

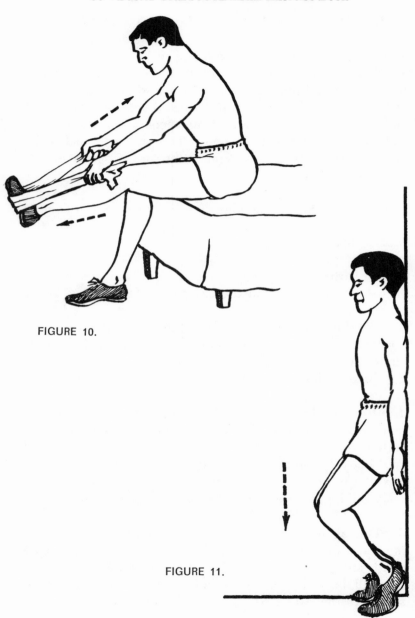

FIGURE 10.

FIGURE 11.

and not to drop down too far. Once down, hold the position for two counts and then slide back up the wall to a standing position (Figure 11).

6. Towel Roll. Spread a towel on the floor before the edge of the bed. Sitting on the bed, place the toes of both feet at the edge of the towel closest to you, and proceed to gather the towel, bit by bit, with your toes, behind your feet until you have gathered and "walked" across the entire towel.

KNEE EXERCISES

Probably the most commonly afflicted of all large joints in arthritis is the knee joint. It is here that people tend to have the worst swelling and pain, often so severe that they are unable to walk. It is essential to regain the ability to bend, extend, rotate and half-bend the knees, for if the knees are stiffened permanently in any position it becomes impossible to walk. The following exercises prevent the deformity from developing, and allow relaxation of stiffness. The exercises also help you regain and maintain strength in the thigh muscles, for these are the main controlling muscles of the knee.

1. Lie on your back with your legs straight. Contract the muscles of your whole leg, all at once. While you do this, tighten your kneecap and try to flatten the knee down on the bed as much as possible. Relax and repeat with the other leg.

2. The Leg Swing. Sit on a high rigid bed or table with your legs hanging over the edge. Be sure your toes cannot touch the floor. Now, slowly raise and lower one foot to a count of four on the way up and four on the way down. Repeat with your other leg. As you become adept at this exercise, you may increase the weight that is being lifted by adding slight weights to your feet, such as sandbags or the metal weights available at orthopedic supply houses (Figure 12).

3. *Knee Raises.* Sit on a bed with your back well supported and your legs straight out in front of you. Slowly slide your foot back on the bed toward your torso, thus raising the knee. Do this to a count of three, and then return the leg, also to a count of three, to the original position. Repeat, as with all of these exercises, with your other leg.

4. *Bicycle.* This exercise should only be done by people who are quite agile, and who do not have severe back problems.

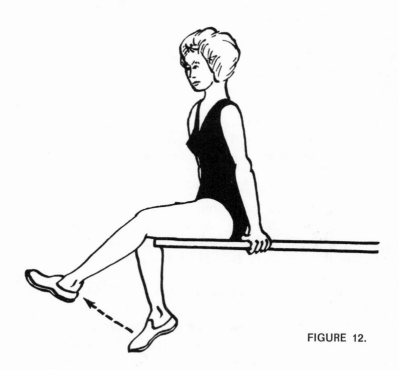

FIGURE 12.

Lie on your back and raise your lower body up in the air, supporting it at the hips with your hands. Bicycle your legs for ten rotations. Reverse the direction for ten more rotations, and then relax.

5. Lie on your stomach on a bed or floor space. Wrap a towel around one ankle, holding onto the ends with both hands, so that your arms are behind your body as you lie on the bed. Try to flex the knees by pulling on the ends of the towel. You should start out by pulling very gently and slowly, and not forcing the knee into too extreme a flexion (Figure 13).

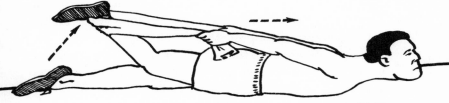

FIGURE 13.

6. _Knee Rotation._ Stand beside a chair with one hand on the back of it for balance. Lift one knee into the air, slightly at first and then higher as you gain increasing agility. Once it is suspended in the air, rotate the bottom of the leg, from the calf down, in a circle, keeping the thigh still and in front of the body. Rotate ten times and then relax. Rotate the other leg.

7. _Modified Passé._ Stand beside a chair with one hand on the back of it for balance. Lift one leg with your knee bent, resting your foot against the calf of the opposite leg. The second step is to swing the lower leg (from the calf down) gently out from the knee toward the side of the room. Hold it for two counts and bring it back. Then slowly lower it to the floor. Repeat this once, and then exercise the alternate leg.

HIP EXERCISES

When afflicted with arthritis the hip, of course, is the most crippling joint, for two reasons. The first is that arthritis of the hip is quite common and extremely painful. The second is that without the use of the hips, the body cannot bear weight, nor can we walk. Often in osteoarthritis of the hip, fusion takes place, thus restricting nearly all hip motion. The hip joint is what we call a "ball and socket" joint. That means that we have a wide range of motion in a hip that is normal. When osteoarthritis sets in, though, many or all of these directional capabilities may be impaired or eliminated. The following exercises are brought together to provide a system which prevents hip deformities. This is done by utilizing muscles which would oppose the development of such deformities. Development of these muscles is very important for lifetime prevention of osteoarthritis of the hip.

1. Lie on your back on your bed or floor. Hold your legs straight up in front of you. Move one approximately fifteen inches to the side and then return it to the side of the other leg. Repeat with the other leg.

2. Leg Raises. Lie on your back, your legs extended in front of you on the bed. Slowly, to a count of four, raise one leg, keeping your knee straight. When you lower, lower it to a count of four also. Repeat with the other leg (Figure 14). After you have raised and lowered each leg, repeat the action—but this time with your knees bent.

3. Backward Leg Raises. Lie on your bed or exercise floor with your face down. Slowly, to a count of three, lift your leg backward, making sure to keep your knee straight. Hold your leg in the position for two counts, and then begin to lower, to a count of three again.

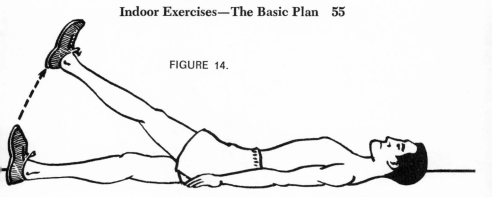

FIGURE 14.

4. Table Leg Swing. Stand beside a sturdy table. Rest the buttock and leg of one side of your body along the edge of the table, allowing the other leg to swing freely. Balancing yourself on the table with both hands placed wherever you feel is best, swing the affected leg back and forth slowly, from the hip, three full times. Repeat with the other leg (Figure 15).

5. Toe Touch. Sit on your bed or floor with your legs extended straight before you. Try to touch your toes with your fingertips. Be sure when you do this exercise to bend forward as far as you can without straining your back, and to keep your trunk rigid.

BACK AND SPINE EXERCISES

Naturally, a big part of rejuvenating the spine is practicing the postural exercises mentioned earlier. However, closer attention to back problems is advised. There are chiropractors and doctors who claim miraculous results from manipulation of the spine. These claims may well be warranted, but these techniques are quite serious and can be dangerous. Any time a remedy involves the spine directly, we must be very careful

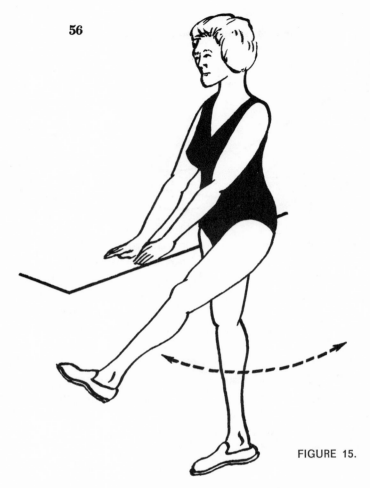

FIGURE 15.

and sure of it, and of the person performing it. Mis-manipulation, even if slight, could cause permanent paralysis. The following exercises are designed to loosen up the stiffness of the spine without involving any serious operations or manipulations. It must be emphasized that all of these exercises should be done in a flowing manner and not jerkily.

1. Stand in the center of the room. Your feet should be about shoulder width apart. Put your hands above your shoulders and clasp your fingers together behind your head. Very slowly, you should arch backward as far as you can go, just from the waist up. Do not *bend* back, or you will be thrown off balance. Then, very slowly bend forward and drop your body from the waist toward your feet. Try to move toward your toes with elbows as you do this. Now, stand up slowly until you are standing straight and then arch back again. Return to a normal standing position.

2. *Side Bend.* Stand with your heels together. Your arms should be at your sides. Slowly, to a count of five, slide one arm down the outside of your thigh toward the knee of that side. Do not push yourself too far so that you are in pain. Resume your normal position, also to a count of five. Repeat the exercise with the other side (Figure 16).

3. *Simple Twists.* Simple twists are the best exercises for this sort of stiffness. Stand in the center of a room, and put your hands at your waist comfortably. Twist the upper part of your body around so that one shoulder points backwards as far as possible. Return to normal position, and then twist in the other direction.

4. *Chair Twist.* Sit erect in a straight-backed chair. Place your hands on top of your head, keeping your elbows back. Your chin should be tucked down and your tummy flat. Keep your chest high, and slowly exhale a little air, thus flattening your upper stomach in the area around the diaphragm; now inhale. Do this five times, and then turn to the side and repeat the exercise as you sit semi-twisted in the chair.

5. Sit or stand comfortably, and bend your neck forward to bring your chin down against your chest. Slowly arch your neck backward as far as it will go. Then, roll it from side to side, bringing each ear down onto a shoulder. Bring your

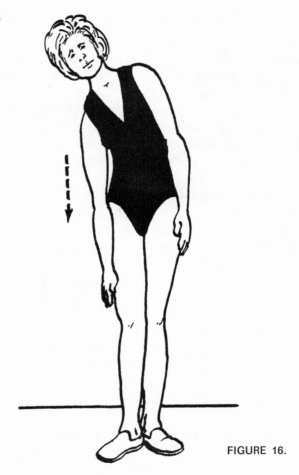

FIGURE 16.

head up again in its normal position, and turn it from side to side, not quickly, but easily. When you have finished this, move your head and neck in a circular motion, making sure that all the joints and muscles are stretched and pulled. When done properly, this exercise should send tiny shivering feelings up the back of your neck and your shoulders. This is also a good exercise to do when you are tense or nervous (Figure 17).

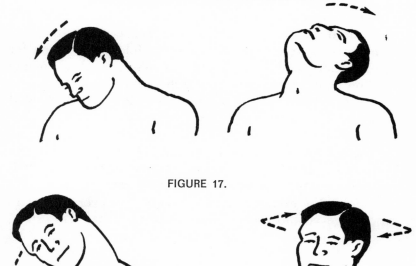

FIGURE 17.

6. This is a final, quieting exercise intended to maintain the movement of the ribs. Stand in the center of the room and take a deep, deep breath, involving both your diaphragm and your ribs. Hold the air for a few seconds, to a count of four, and then release, very slowly, also to a count of four.

7. *The Cradle.* Sit down on the floor, and with your knees bent and together, clasp your hands under your knees and roll back on your spine, then back to a sitting position. You should do this very carefully, so that you do not lose control and roll back too far. The exercise is to be done in one rolling motion, back and forth, resting momentarily everytime you return to the original position. Do this five times, or start at two and work up to five.

8. *The Cat.* Kneel on the floor, in a cat or dog fashion. Lift your head upwards, stretching your throat and at the same time curving your back downwards. Hold the position for three counts, and then slowly and gently, with a flowing motion, lower your head and arch your back up as far as possible. If your eyes are open, you should be seeing behind you when you do this exercise.

These exercises are the foundation of the program. Once you start, it is essential to do your program each day. Obviously on certain days you will feel more energetic and more like doing the exercises than on others. However, I want to encourage you to exercise particularly on the "lazy" days, because these are the days when you will most need to be limbered.

In addition to the basic plan, I think it is a good idea to choose at least one exercise from the chapter on yoga exercises. These are enormously helpful in stretching and thus relaxing stiff joints.

Following these, in Chapter 5, are several suggestions for exercises outside of the home. These are, of course, only to be added after you have passed several weeks successfully and consistently limbering up your body through the basic plan.

CHAPTER FOUR

SPECIAL YOGA EXERCISES FOR YOUR ARTHRITIC PROBLEMS

For centuries yoga has been used in the Orient for health purposes as well as religious ones. Only in the last couple of decades, though, has it become popular in our country. I find many yoga exercises excellent for limbering my body and for keeping my muscles supple. Another great benefit of yoga exercises is that they are very calming. Performing the soothing stretches of muscle-elongating yoga positions is always a good way to complete your exercise periods. For several years now I have assimilated a group of yoga positions into my daily exercise routine, and I find them to be extremely helpful. Yoga exercises, besides being good limbering tools, are excellent toners for your muscles. I know several professional dancers who practice yoga for anywhere from half an hour to an hour every day, in addition to their dancing. They claim that the yoga keeps their muscles toned so that they respond more quickly when at work dancing.

People who have tried my exercise program have had excellent results with the yoga exercises. The yoga works for many elderly patients as well as the other exercises, because yoga is based on very slow movements and older people seem to enjoy and benefit as much if not more from these as from other, more strenuous exercises.

Alice, an elderly friend of mine, had been teaching classics in a San Francisco university for more than fifty years when I met her. I was giving a lecture at her school a couple of years ago on the subject of nutrition and exercise as being just as important to good health as a proper mental state. After I had delivered my speech, she came up to the lectern and began asking me several pointed questions about the material I had just presented concerning exercise and good health. She did not mention her arthritis, but she did ask me very abruptly what I expected older people whose joints had stiffened to do about getting enough exercise. If I really believed in physical fitness for everyone, she said, then it was my commitment and my responsibility to develop a program of exercises that older people could follow.

I admired Alice's forthrightness and her spunk. She did not mince words about what she expected. And though she had not mentioned it, as she stood before me it became apparent that she suffered from arthritis, for I could see the knobbed, deformed finger joints of her hands as she moved them confidently while she spoke.

I invited her to lunch with me, and at first she declined, claiming that she was much too busy to dawdle over lunch—that she had papers to grade and lectures to prepare, and that she never ate lunch without doing work simultaneously. At this time, this energetic little lady was nearing seventy-five years of age.

After intense coaxing on my part, she agreed to our luncheon date. We ate in the school cafeteria, where I was amazed at the number of students who could not pass her table without saying hello. Alice was clearly one of the best-loved teachers at the university. We spoke at length of the problems of the elderly whose limbs and joints had stiffened too much to exercise properly. When I told her about the system of arthritis exercises I had developed, she quickly explained that exercises were one thing, but exercises that an older person might try were something else again, indeed. At this point it seemed futile to try to convince her of the feasibility of such a program for herself, so I brought up the subject of yoga. Alice brightened immediately as I explained certain of the stretches to her.

She began the program that evening and continued working with yoga for several weeks. Little by little she added certain exercises from the rest of the plan to her combination of yoga exercises. Shortly after I left San Francisco and arrived back home in the Southwest, I received a note from her that reported much progress, particularly in loosening up her shoulders and her spine. The last time I saw her she explained to me that she does her exercises faithfully each morning before leaving for the university, and that she's able to lecture to all of her classes and to keep her office hours in the afternoon without her back beginning to pinch or ache in the slightest.

Alice, like so many other elderly people, was enchanted by the fluidity and slow, graceful pace of yoga exercises. The basic principle behind yoga as regards stiffness is that a supple body allows energy to flow freely throughout the body, and consequently, that stiff joints block this flow and sap energy from your body. A stiff body, then, it is believed, causes all sorts of ills and pains. The purpose of these yoga movements is to restore the elasticity to your limbs and joints through very controlled, very slow self-manipulation of one's body, with great emphasis on one's joints. Yoga is very good to begin a program of exercise with, because it diminishes much of the initial strain and pain which an arthritic will feel when he is first beginning an exercise program. The manipulation involved here is mild, and these slow-motion movements, particularly the position holds, are able to reach down deep into your joints, relieving the stiffness.

You should not be at all discouraged if you are not able to wrap yourself into all sorts of intricate positions like those which I am sure you have seen on television. That is not the goal of this system of exercise. We want to limber your joints and stiffened muscles, and this elasticity *always* comes little by little, yet, with continued use of these exercises, it does always come. The principle is that you hold a position for increasingly longer periods of time each time you perform it. Day by day, you will be able to hold the position longer, and without even realizing it, your position itself will become more advanced. But at first, if you can move an inch and hold the position for five seconds, you are already beginning to move and to manipulate your body; already you have taken a step toward your goal of relief from the pain of arthritis, and this step will grow larger each day.

I would like to emphasize that this is exactly how you should begin your program. You should think in terms of *inches*. In any exercise you choose, you should only move until you experience some discomfort. At this point, you should *hold the position for a count of five*, and then relax. Try to repeat the exercise two or three times. Each day, try to move only an *inch* farther and to hold the position only *one* second longer. You should never perform an exercise to the point where it causes you pain.

It is natural that some days you will be unable to practice at all because of pain. This is to be expected. On these days, you should try the breathing exercise described in the previous chapter, to keep your muscles freshened, but you should not attempt yoga or any other exercises on these days. When the intense pain has subsided, then you can continue your program of exercise. It is to be emphasized that relieving the stiffness and the pain of arthritis can never be achieved in one fell swoop, or even in a completely straight line. Bad and painful periods are part and parcel of the illness, and a few steps of progress coupled with one step backward is not unnatural, nor should you be discouraged when this occurs.

The following exercises, as indicated above, should be performed two or three times, and should be held for anywhere from a count of five to ten, five being a fine beginning goal.

It is also important after you have held your position for the required amount of time that you do not spring out of it quickly. Everything in yoga is in slow motion, and you should take as much time unwinding from the position as you took in achieving it.

1. The Leg Pull. Sit with your legs extended straight before you. Your back should be straight up as you begin this exercise. Clasp your hands on your legs just below your knees, rounding your back slightly as you do so. Now, to a count of five, bend slightly forward, pulling your trunk toward your knees. Obviously, one who suffers from arthritis cannot be expected to pull himself all the way down so that his face is touching his knees, but you should attempt to pull as far toward this goal as possible without straining. Remember, an inch, if that is all you can manage, is sufficient (Figure 18).

2. The Alternating Leg Pull. This exercise, along with the previous one, is a marvelous limberer for arthritic joints in the legs and back. As with the Leg Pull, sit with your legs stretched straight out before you. Slowly bring your right heel up the inside of your left leg, lodging it as far up as you

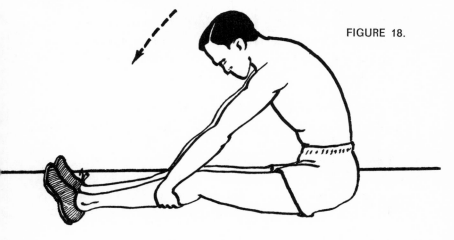

FIGURE 18.

can get it without too much discomfort. Now, again slowly, reach your arms and hands up toward the ceiling and lean slightly backwards. Again, very slowly, bend forward and take a firm hold on your left leg or ankle, depending on how much you can stretch at this point. Being sure not to strain, gently pull your trunk downward toward your legs as far as possible. At this movement, your elbows should be bending outward. Now, release the tension from your neck by letting it go limp. Hold this position, without moving, for a count of five, or less if the strain is too great. Repeat with your other leg.

3. *The Cobra.* This exercise also is good for limbering stiff and painful back joints. This is a modified version of the one normally used by people who practice yoga, and this is specifically designed for arthritic patients. Lie on your stomach comfortably, with your hands and arms resting straight at your sides. Your legs should be straight also. Put your hands, palms down, on the floor next to your shoulders, so that your elbows are bent outward. Very slowly, to a count of five, push up with your arms until your trunk is raised off of the floor. Normally, the goal would be a deep arc of your back, but here the goal is simply to limber your spine, and so whatever movement you can make short of straining yourself is acceptable. When you are elevated as far as you can go, hold the position for five seconds and then slowly lower yourself (Figure 19).

4. *Toe and Foot Exercise.* This exercise begins while you are in a sitting position on the floor. You should be sitting with your legs tucked under you—"sitting on your haunches" is what we used to call it, but you should not be putting your weight back onto your feet. Instead, place your fingertips on the floor beside your hips, and let the weight of your body rest on your fingers. Depending upon how advanced your

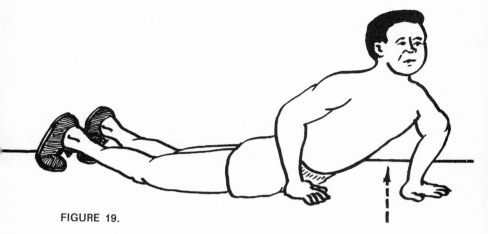

FIGURE 19.

arthritis is, it will probably be quite difficult to do anything else. Now, very slowly lower your buttocks onto your heels. (Your weight should be resting on the balls of the feet, heels off the floor if possible. If not, then rest your feet flat upon the floor.) With your hands in this position of support, you can control completely the amount of weight that you loose upon your feet. Once you have applied as much weight as possible without undue strain, hold the position from one to twenty seconds (Figure 20).

5. *The Twist.* This is another spinal exercise, but unlike the Leg Pull, which concentrates on outward bending of the spine, and unlike the Cobra, which concentrates on inward bending of the spine, the Twist works on achieving a spiral twisting movement. In this exercise, the "locks" and "stretches" which form the basis of yogic movements are clearly seen. The thigh locks the lumbar area of the back so that the middle and upper areas may twist and stretch against this lock. This is the quickest and most efficient spine loosener of any yoga exercises.

To execute the Twist, sit on the floor with your legs ex-

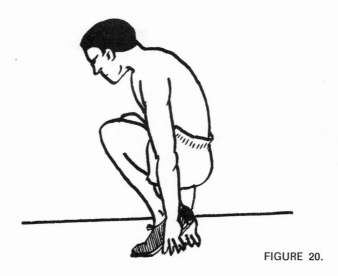

FIGURE 20.

tended out before you. Place your right sole firmly against the upper inside of your left thigh, or as near to it up your leg as you can get it. Bring your extended left leg up, bending the knee, and slip it over your right leg, placing the left foot firmly on the floor. At this point, your balance may become impaired, so take your left hand and place it firmly on the floor behind you. Also, straighten your right leg out. This is a modification of the full twisting exercise done by yogis, but it is quite enough twist for anyone suffering from arthritis. When you have regained your balance and you feel comfortable with the position, slowly twist your trunk and head as far to your *left* as possible. When you have twisted around, hold the position for five counts, and then slowly return. Be sure to unwind as cautiously and as slowly as you moved getting into this complex exercise. I realize that there are many parts to the Twist and that you might not be able to execute all of them at once. A good goal for the first time you try this exercise is simply the first movement of it. If you can bend your leg partway up the inside of your other leg and hold it there for a few seconds, this is as good a start as anyone could ask for. In subsequent trials, attempt the other parts of the exercise, until eventually you can put all the parts together at the same time.

6. *Postural.* This exercise helps loosen the spine and back, as well as the shoulders and neck. It is a good, all-around posture balancing exercise. Stand erect in the center of your exercise space, with your feet slightly apart. Raise your arms slowly, until they are straight out before you at shoulder height. Place your hands together, palms down. Very slowly, turn your torso ninety degrees to your left, without moving the feet. While you do this you should make an effort to keep your eyes on your hands. In this way, your neck and head turn with you. Hold the side position for a count of five, and then slowly return. Be sure to complete the exercise by again dropping your hands to your sides.

7. *The Neck Twist.* This exercise is invaluable in relieving tension and stiffness in your neck joints and muscles, and it has the added attraction that it can be performed almost anywhere. Place your elbows on a level surface (a floor, a table, a desk, etc.). Your elbows should be fairly close together and your arms should be parallel. Place your head between your hands, cupping your ears with the palms of your hands. Gently drop your head forward a bit, until you can clasp your hands on the lower back of your head. Push down with your hands very slowly until your chin touches your chest, or as far as you can push without discomfort. Close your eyes and hold this position for a count of five. Do not move your arms or unbend your elbows, but turn your head slowly and rest your chin in your left arm. Grip the back of your head firmly with your right hand. Turn your head very slowly as far as you can to your left, keeping your eyes closed. Hold this position for a count of five. Do not move your elbows or arms, but turn your head in the opposite direction, reversing the action (resting chin on right arm) and holding this third position for a count of five again. Resume the original position and bow your head against the flat surface for a moment to release the energy of the movement.

8. The Knee Stretch. This exercise allows the knees and thighs to bend outward, and it is important because this movement is a stretch that is generally not performed during the day's activities. Consequently, for the arthritic it is quite important to loosen the knees in this way, because he or she will hardly ever get the chance to do it otherwise. Sit erect on the floor and place the soles of your feet together, as far out before you as is necessary for comfort. While keeping your back straight, bring your feet as far toward you as possible, and place your clasped hands around your feet if you can bring them in far enough to comfortably get hold of your feet. This is the first movement of the exercise, and for the seriously afflicted arthritic, it may be, at first, all that the sufferer can accomplish. If this is the case with you, hold the position for a count of five and then release. In ensuing days, you will be able to perform the second half, and you will also be able to pull your legs and feet farther in toward your body.

The second part of the exercise is as follows: With your hands clasped around your feet, pull up on them and allow your knees to press gently as far toward the floor as possible. Hold this position for a count of five and then relax your legs so that they come upward and rest.

9. The Leg Clasp. This exercise has two main benefits. The first is that it loosens up stiff leg muscles, and the second is that it loosens stiff shoulder joints and also works to loosen your spine. You should begin the exercise from a standing position. Bend forward ever so slightly, and extend your arms until they point outward over your toes. This is not a major extension, but simply to get you started on the main part of the movement. Bend forward very slowly and bring your trunk down toward the floor as far as possible without straining. While you are doing this be careful not to bend your knees. Clasp your hands behind your knees or calves, at whatever point is most comfortable for you. Now, very gently pull your trunk as far toward your knees as possible without strain. Hold this position for a count of five without moving. Allow your trunk to rise slowly from its bent over position, making sure that you count at least five counts while you are coming up.

I want to emphasize that in any yoga exercise, it is not necessary to try for maximum stretch during the first week you are doing the exercise. Yoga is unlike any other kind of exercise in that once you have achieved a certain amount of flexibility with yoga, you will never lose it. So don't be in a hurry to be able to perform these exercises perfectly. When you master one level of stretch, you will keep it for as long as you practice the exercises. There is no rush, for you have only to do a little each day to achieve greater elasticity and to relieve the pain.

CHAPTER FIVE

MAKING THE MOST OF YOUR DAILY SITUATIONS

Now that I have presented the basic exercise plan to you, it is essential to move to the subject of everyday life. Obviously, beginning an exercise program is a big step on its own. However, it is only part of an overall plan. If you have been sedentary because of the pain and stiffness caused by arthritis, you will want now to change that lifestyle. You will, over a period of weeks, develop new freedom of movement, and your old way of life simply will not accommodate the things you will be able to do. Consequently, it is important to examine how you can put small changes into those things you do each day.

As I explained earlier in regard to posture, arthritics frequently find themselves having to adjust to pain, having to change their lives for the pain. Just as we saw that posture is thrown out of balance to relieve the pain of arthritis, so we now see that daily life itself has often been altered to accommodate one's disease.

Oftentimes people eliminate certain activities from their daily lives. Walking, for instance, is often the first to go. And of course, all sports activities are usually cut from people's lives simply on principle. A housewife who suffers from arthritis will necessarily create many shortcuts in her work, some of which may even call for skipping certain more strenuous and difficult activities, such as moving furniture to clean under it. A man in an office situation will do the same, too. He will avoid walking from one end of his office to the other, or moving files, or sitting too long at his desk.

All of these things are understandable modifications of daily life for an arthritic. Yet most of them are ultimately unnecessary. Certainly one must alter one's life, but there are ways to do it which are not merely accommodating, but which are beneficial and help you progress toward relief from your condition. In other words, it is better to perform your daily activities, perhaps in a slightly modified way, but with a goal in mind of using them as aids to health and mobility rather than as simply impossibly painful chores of daily life.

A THERAPEUTIC HOME SITUATION

It may seem contradictory to advocate rest in a book about exercise as a relief for arthritis. However, a prescribed amount of rest during the day is not synonymous with inactivity. It also does not always mean rest in bed.

Rest periods can incorporate a variety of positions. Rest is indeed an essential treatment for inflamed and painful joints, and at least an hour a day should be spent relaxing the particular arthritic areas of your body. This rest should be taken when you are finished with your daily routine, so that your mind is cleared of petty annoyances.

If your knees or feet are the arthritic joints, then sit in a chair with your legs propped in a comfortable position and read or knit or watch television for the hour. If your hands and elbows are painful, this same position may suffice for that malady.

If your back or shoulders are afflicted, you probably should lie down on a bed or couch that is comfortable, but that is not too soft or malleable. This would seem to be the best way to rest these joints.

Be sure that you get one *solid* hour of rest; that is, one hour when the arthritic joints are not required to support any weight, and when they are not being used at all. You can decide best for yourself when and where you might find the time to accomplish this.

As regards rest, it is important to receive *proper* rest, which means proper posture and vehicles for rest. For lying down (and this is important to note in terms of sleep, too), a proper bed is essential. Resting for an hour on a bed which strains your back is harmful. Most beds are too soft, so that when you lie on the mattress your spine is allowed to curve with the mattress. This aggravates arthritic problems, and you will arise from your rest *un*relaxed and frequently with a backache.

To correct this problem, a bedboard of one-half to three-quarter-inch plywood which covers the full length and width of the bed should be placed between the mattress and the springs to give proper support and to maintain the spine in its proper position. The bedboard also is valuable in that it prevents flexion or bending of hip joints while you are lying on your back. This sort of bed will often cause discomfort for the first few nights, but most people find that consistent use of such a bed diminishes pain and fatigue considerably after four or five days.

Another aspect of a proper bed is proper height. It is much easier to get up from a bed that is higher than normal beds, than from one that is lower. I advise raising your bed about six inches from its present height. This can be done by putting six-inch blocks under each of the casters. In this way, you will not be forced to stoop, strain, or bend, which requires using many of your joints in awkward ways, to perform the otherwise simple task of getting out of bed. Many arthritics are discouraged the first moment they awake in the morning because they realize that they must perform the simple but excruciating task of getting out of bed. This discouragement, as well as the pain, can be eliminated by raising the bed.

The other major form of rest, *chair rest*, should also be carefully approached. A chair, like the bed, should also be raised from the floor from four to six inches. In this way your toes and the balls of your feet should just touch the floor, rather than being scrunched against the floor. The seat of your chair should be flat, and the back should be broad and high, and uncurved. You should always sit in the chair with your buttocks touching the back of it. This position eliminates slumping, which puts a painful strain on your back rather than affording the quick comfort you might seem to derive at first.

In conducting yourself through daily life, you should keep in mind that pain is to be avoided. Pain is a good indicator that something is not quite right, that your posture is bad or that you have been straining too much. In addition, when you feel painful, you are draining your strength and energy. So, a housewife who has a load of ironing to do will naturally want to get it out of the way, and do it all at once. No one wants to keep thinking about a stack of wrinkled clothes, when you can do them all at one time and be done with the task. However, standing over an ironing board and lifting a heavy iron again and again for two or three hours is a certain way to cause yourself much pain and fatigue.

However much you want to finish your housework all at once, remember that avoidance of pain and fatigue about your joints is more important. It is much wiser to iron for half an hour to an hour at a time and then rest or go to some activity that uses other parts of your body, and then return to ironing later.

PLANNING YOUR DAY

One of the basic points to remember is that you should *never do one activity for too long a time*. Home workers are lucky in this respect, for they can do their work in whatever order they choose. This rule also applies to forms of entertainment in the home, such as television. Our daily habits usually include several hours of television a day, and this is certainly too long a period to be sitting or lying down at any one time. When the arthritic sits for several hours in front of a television set, he becomes even stiffer than usual in his arthritic joints. The solution to this is not to cut out television. Deprivation of this sort will never solve the problem. Rather, one should watch television, or perform another similar activity, for short periods of time.

Another point to remember during your daily activities is that any motion can have two-fold value. It can be functional as well as therapeutic. Anytime you stand before an ironing board, you should be standing straight and tall, almost as though you were performing on a stage. The periods of time spent standing can then be used for postural exercises as well as simply toiling time over the ironing board. When you move your arm back and forth over the board, you should move it in smooth gliding motions, and not jerkily, for this will serve as wrist and elbow joint exercise, as well as simply ironing.

Bending and stooping are prime fatiguers of housewives, and yet they are necessary and continual actions. These movements seem to be the most aggravating to arthritis. Many women complain to me that they are fine until they begin to pick up their family's clothes or their children's toys, and at this point everything begins to ache. This could not be more significant. Bending over twenty times a day or more not only strains the back and shoulders, but a constant grabbing motion also pulls at the joints of your hands and arms. A good way to avoid this pain and fatigue, and to transform this action into a beneficial one, is to practice a different form of bending.

First practice this new bending with the aid of a chair. Stand beside the back of a chair with your hand resting gently on the top of it for support. Slowly bend at your knees until you have descended far enough so that you might pick up an imaginary piece of clothing. Now, while going down was the easy part, lifting yourself back up may be a bit harder. The weight, though, should fall to your thigh muscles. It may take a while before you become adept at this, to the point where you will be able to do it and retain your balance on your own without the aid of a chair. However, this type of bending is an essential thing to learn and to cultivate as a habitual way of reaching to the floor. It has several advantages. Your spine is not strained or twisted. This is particularly important if you are lifting anything heavy. The second advantage is that the strain is on your leg *muscles* and not so much on a joint of any kind. In this way, you will develop healthy leg muscles. The third advantage is that your knee joints will receive extra exercise. Once you learn to bend this way, I am confident that you, like so many other people, will find yourself and your joints less tired and less painful at the day's end.

Another kind of action-transformation you can perform is that of sweeping or vacuuming. In both cases you should employ only smooth, fluid movements, and you should not try to stretch beyond reasonable capacity. Start out by treating these actions as exercises, *i.e.*, by using small, graceful movements. If you have to take a few more steps because your range of motion is smaller, this is still advisable. It is better to move your body in small motions at first, rather than to make wide, swinging movements, which will ultimately cause you pain and more fatigue than necessary. This is a very important point. In altering your daily activities and work in this way, you will be saving yourself from what probably has become normal pain and fatigue.

A THERAPEUTIC OFFICE SITUATION

Just as the basic rule for the home situation was never to do any one thing for too long a period of time, so it is the rule for the office situation. If you are an office worker who sits at a desk all day, this is harder to accomplish. Certainly you should shift your sitting position as much as possible. If you happen to have a private office within which you work, you will be able to take frequent breaks from sitting, simply by standing up and walking around the room. The basic exercises outlined earlier in the book which required you to stand in the middle of the room and stretch, can be done in such a situation, and this is very strongly advised. To stand in the center of the room and perform these relaxing mild exercises every three hours would not be too frequent, and would help you greatly in terms of losing your fatigue and strain. Remember, strain and fatigue cause pain, and it is important to do all we can to relieve these problems.

If you do not have an office or a situation where you can easily and conveniently change your position, or practice these breathing and stretching exercises, there are still many ways you can modify and use your work situation to deal with the arthritic condition.

If you are, for example, a secretary, you must naturally spend a great amount of your day sitting and typing. An important thing to remember here is never to sit except in the correct postural position, with your back straight and your feet flat on the floor. Be sure you avoid crossing your legs or ankles, because this not only locks your joints into unnatural positions, but it cuts off circulation to your limbs. As often as possible you should stand up and stretch. Try to break up the typing and the sitting with various other duties, like filing or xeroxing, so that you will not be typing for long stretches at a time. If you must sit when you are not typing, try to sit in

different places and positions so that your joints do not become stiffly locked into any one mold.

If you must stand for long periods, be sure to stand solidly
on both feet. It is important not to delegate the entire weight
of your body to one foot or the other, for this puts undue
strain on knee and hip joints, thus aggravating an arthritic
condition.

A good exercise to do while you are driving in the car on
the way to or from work is as follows: Grip the steering wheel
with both hands, your arms extended, at the nine o'clock and
three o'clock positions. Exert pressure on the wheel, your
hands pressing toward each other, as though you wanted to
bend or crush the steering wheel. Hold this position for five
seconds. Relax. Now, with your hands in the same position
try to pull the wheel back into shape. Hold for five seconds
and then relax. It is, of course, important while you are performing this exercise that the car be stopped at a stop light,
or perhaps perform it while you are waiting for the car to
warm up.

Another exercise that can be done any time and any place
is the Shoulder Hunch. First, sit up straight and shake your
shoulders and neck slowly and gently to release any accum-
ulated tension. Then slowly "hunch" your shoulders, draw-
ing them up toward your ears. Hold them tightly in this
position for five seconds and then release them and relax.
This exercise may be repeated three times at the most for
a start.

A third exercise which will greatly benefit people who
suffer from arthritis, is called Chest Expansion. This, too, can
be done most any time and any place. Stand up from your
desk or work area, making sure you have enough room for a
complete extension of your arms. Your hands and arms should
begin this exercise at your side. Slowly raise them to the side,
bending your elbows, until they are perpendicular to the line

of your body; at this point your elbows should be turned out at either side. Your arms should be at shoulder height. Slowly stretch them out before you, and as you do this, make sure you feel the full stretch and extension of your joints. Now, bring your arms directly back as far as possible, trying to keep them in line with your shoulders. When you can go no farther, drop your arms so that you can clasp your hands behind you. Always, when doing this exercise, try to keep as erect as possible through your trunk area, and do not bend forward.

The second part of this exercise is to bend back very slowly, keeping your arms and hands in the backward, clenched position. Be sure that when you bend back you do so only very slightly, without straining your back or shoulders. Slowly resume your original position, still keeping your hands clasped behind your back.

The third and last movement is to bend forward, also very slowly, as far as you can without straining or losing your balance. Hold the exercise in each position for a count of five, and move to each position to a count of five. Finally, resume your basic position to standing with your arms at your sides.

A good exercise for secretaries and other people who must sit in one position for most of the day is the Simple Twist. Sit with your back erect and your buttocks pushed as far back in the chair as they will go. Your arms should be at your sides and your feet flat on the floor. Cross your right leg over your left and let it rest comfortably in this position. Hold fast to the seat of the chair with your right hand. Cross your left arm over your right knee and let it grip gently upon your left knee. As you remain in this position, gripping the seat of the chair and holding your left knee firmly, slowly twist as far as you can to your right. Hold this position for a count of five, and then slowly turn back to your original position. Repeat the twist once more and then resume the basic position, uncrossing your arms and legs. Perform this exercise to the other side, twice, as you did with the first side.

The last exercise for your office situation is the Neck Roll. This is a good exercise to do at least twice a day, whether or not you have arthritis in your shoulders or back. This is a relaxing and refreshing practice. Sit erect in a chair, your head held straight and comfortably. Slowly bend your head forward and let your chin rest against your chest. Hold this position for a count of five. Next, slowly roll and twist your head to the extreme left. Hold this also for a count of five. Slowly roll and twist your head to the extreme backward position. In this position you should be able to feel your chin and throat muscles stretching. Hold this also for five counts. Slowly roll and twist your head to the extreme right, and hold for five counts. *Your eyes should be closed during the entire exercise.* You can repeat the movements once or twice, until you have loosened any tightness and the tension has been drained away.

Each of these exercises can be performed once or twice daily in most office situations. As a matter of fact, many of my arthritic friends find that when the office workers see them performing these exercises and when they see how much more relaxed and refreshed and full of energy the people are once they have finished with the exercises, the whole office participates in the exercise period. The amazing thing about these exercises is that they can do so much for your well-being and yet they are not time-consuming; they are fairly simple and refreshing. Unfortunately, most office situations cannot be altered as we would like them to be, yet with the use of these simple exercises, you can modify the environment and your daily work routine so as to take much of the strain and fatigue from your work hours.

CHAPTER SIX

STAYING ACTIVE OUT-OF-DOORS

Now that you have begun your exercise program and, I am sure, are feeling the benefits of your new mobility, it is important to think in terms of developing new out-of-doors activities which, up to now, you probably considered too strenuous. Oftentimes the person suffering from arthritis will simply learn to live without any kind of outdoor pastimes. I have friends who always used to refuse my suggestions of swimming dates or picnics, because they claimed that they couldn't abide all that moving around.

This attitude, while understandable when you have been in extreme pain from arthritic joints, is very unhealthy and unnecessary. Unhealthy, because shying away from sports leads one to hide from any sort of outdoor activity, and eventually from the outdoors itself. This is an important psychological point. For example, a woman who declines a swimming date or a game of golf because her arthritic joints are bothering her will probably replace that activity with one of an indoor sort. In her mind, she will begin to see indoor pastimes as replacing outdoor ones, until it will become more a habit for her to "hide" from the sunlight and fresh air than any actual need. I have seen this happen time and again. People will end up leading sedentary lives, out of the sun, away from the sky and the trees. They confine themselves, like moles, to the four walls of their homes, and to the musty air within. This is fatal to a human being. We were meant to get fresh air and to walk in the sunlight beneath the trees.

It is totally unnecessary for an arthritis sufferer to end up confined to his or her home. This again is an example of the vicious circle. The more you hide from outdoor exercise, the harder it is to do it. Of course, I am not suggesting a rousing set of tennis, but there are more moderate types of exercise which can be performed, which are vital to your life. I also find that being outside has a distinct psychological effect on people. The more time they spend outside, the more capable they feel they are, and indeed the more capable they become. This also means that the happier they become, for self-esteem is a major contributor to a happy individual.

I have a friend who is a mechanic. He's not very old (I believe he is in his early thirties), yet a year or so ago he became afflicted with arthritis in his knees. The first time I discovered his condition, I had gone to his garage to check on my car, and I saw him working on it *sitting down*. I was a little taken aback when I walked into his work area and saw this, but then he explained to me about his arthritis. It was then that I realized how unhealthy he looked, in general. His skin was pasty and his eyes were glassy-looking. He had seemed quite morose in the last few months, and when I asked him about this he explained that hiking had been his life's love, but since he had been afflicted with arthritis he had not been able to go out into the woods on weekends. I could see how this hobby might have been hampered by his arthritic condition, so I asked him what he did instead to pass the time on Saturday and Sunday, and he replied that he usually watched television and had a few beers.

It was just as I had suspected. Instead of replacing the outdoor activity with another one, he had succumbed to sitting inside his house all weekend. I suggested that we go swimming together on the next Saturday afternoon, but he replied that it would be too painful for him. It was then that I explained to him my interest in arthritis, and the exercise program that I had developed in the last couple of years. He was very interested, and together we worked out an exercise plan for him.

About a month later I took my wife's car in for some minor repairs, and my friend looked very much healthier and happier as he greeted me. He related that he had been practicing the exercises every day, faithfully, and that he had found in them an immense amount of relief from his pain. He also told me that he had taken my suggestion to swim, and had been swimming each weekend since he began the exercises. The outdoor activity, he said, gave him much pleasure. As a matter of fact, he had begun walking again—only a short walk in the afternoon sunshine, but still it was a walk, whereas before he had not imagined that he was capable of walking with his knees in the condition they were in.

This is just one example of someone who felt he must cut himself off from life because of his arthritic condition. This is not at all the case: people who suffer from arthritis are capable of participating in many moderate sports.

First of all, it is good to set aside a time each week, apart from your normal exercise period, when you go outside and do some further exercise of a sporting or leisure nature. If you are afflicted so badly that you cannot even move, I would advise merely setting up a chair in the sunlight in your backyard or on your porch or even next to an open window. It is of the utmost importance merely to be out in the open air. You can sit back in the chair and lean your head back, turning your face to the sun and soaking in the healing rays of nature.

If, however, you are able to do more strenuous activity, there are several with which you might begin. In all of these cases, it is not essential to do an activity which will exercise the arthritic joints of your body. Your indoor exercises are designed for that purpose. The goal here is to use that new-found flexibility and mobility by getting outside, becoming a more active person and, put simply, having a good time. *Be good to yourself.* Don't coop yourself up inside the house, but get out and do something you enjoy. You deserve it!

Probably the easiest activity available to all of us is walking. It takes no long-range plans, equipment, or partners simply to get up from a chair and go outside for a walk. Yet this is perhaps the most neglected of exercises. We build our lives in this society to avoid walking. We drive from place to place, get out of the car and go into a building, do whatever business we have, get back in the car, and drive home. I even know people who *drive* to the corner market. This couldn't be more unhealthy, yet to change this practice we must change our entire way of living and attitudes toward life.

First of all, the basic piece of advice is: *Never ride when you can walk.* This in itself will make a world of difference in your health situation. If you want to go to a shopping center to buy nails for a carpentry project, or to match yarn for a sweater you are knitting, chances are the distance is not more than a mile from your home. A mile is not that great a distance. It is merely several blocks, blocks which might be more interesting to you if you walked them rather than drove right by them. Your neighborhood might take on a completely new perspective in your mind if you walk around it. Too often we learn *not* to look at things, as we drive by them in the car, and we miss much of life that way. So get out in the air and among people whenever you can. *Never ride when you can walk.*

Secondly, a walk once a day just for the purpose of walking can and should become a regular event. I always like to go out for a turn around the neighborhood in the early evening, just before we sit down to dinner. This is a very good time for working people, because it is usually a free time, and it is also a calm time outdoors. Most of the cars are off the streets, people are relaxing, and it is usually an hour when you will be able to free yourself of all your day's petty annoyances. What better way to interact with the people of your community than to walk casually and slowly through the streets passing a few friendly words with your neighbors?

Walks are good anytime the weather is mild. Whatever time you choose, though, you should not walk in intense heat, and you should always walk at a leisurely pace. Outdoor exercise should not seem like a chore. You should not be hopelessly winded when you arrive back home. It is enough that you are out in the fresh air walking about; you do not have to keep a brisk and tiring pace at the same time. Start your walking program by devoting perhaps fifteen minutes to a leisurely walk around the block. After you have done that for a week or so, you might try setting out for half an hour. This pastime, coupled with your new determination to *never ride when you can walk*, will quickly bring a more vibrant glow to your face and a healthier, more active outlook to your life.

Beyond this simple change, there are other more controlled kinds of outdoor exercise you might begin to participate in. First, though, I want to give a very important warning: *Take it easy!* Now that you are exercising each day and have gained a certain amount of mobility, you will be feeling much better and more active. You will want to get out and do all the things you have been depriving yourself of for so long. But let me repeat: *Take it easy.* Do not overdo it at first. You have lots of time to catch up with all the things you've wanted to do for so long.

Swimming is certainly *the* most therapeutic kind of activity available to anyone with arthritis. Water has long been known to be a powerful source of healing, because it serves as a buoy to painful limbs and joints. When you submerge yourself in water, you float. The pressure, strain, and weight are taken off all your painful joints. Consequently, you can move about and get exercise without putting unnecessary strain on your limbs. The contraction and stretching of your muscles in water increase the circulation throughout your body, giving you a feeling of well-being.

Naturally, it is very important that any swimming you do be done in a heated pool. Cold water will always tend to make your muscles and joints stiffen up. Just as hot water therapy does wonders for loosening stiff joints, so does swimming in a warm pool perform much the same job. It should be noted that under no circumstances should an arthritic undertake to swim in the ocean. This could be disastrous, not simply in terms of the cold ocean water, but also because of strong wave action and undertow currents. People who don't have a terribly high level of muscle strength should by no means attempt it.

When you first undertake a swimming session, I suggest that you start out by simply performing some uncomplicated exercises in the shallow end of the pool, letting your body become accustomed to being suspended in water. Only later on should you try to perform actual strokes along the length of the pool.

Remember also, that you should set yourself a time limit of perhaps fifteen minutes to a half an hour, and then stick to that limit. It is all too easy in the buoyancy of the water of a swimming pool not to notice the time fly by, and not to notice how truly tired you are becoming. If you are not careful, you are liable to end up passing the better part of an afternoon in a pool not noticing the time zip past, and consequently waking up the next day with joints aching worse than before. Again, don't overdo it.

Another good form of exercise, but one for the more advanced, is that of hiking. I don't mean by this the strenuous and exhausting hobby of mountain-climbing. Again, hiking can be taken to dangerous extremes. However, a brisk walk through the woods is often refreshing and enjoyable.

An outdoor exercise I would recommend for the more

advanced is bicycle riding. This is an excellent way to keep limber all joints of your legs and feet. But it should be carefully controlled as a pastime, because it can be harmful to those with arthritis of the hip and of the back. If you are able to sit on a bicycle comfortably, though, a bike ride once a day is an excellent way to maintain elasticity in your joints. It is also a good way to develop muscle strength in your legs. Obviously, one of the more important aspects of outdoor exercise is that it gives you a chance, while you are enjoying yourself, to build increased muscular strength. This is vitally important to your recovery, because the stronger you are, the more you will be able to move around, and the more you will want to move around. And obviously, the more mobility you achieve, the less tendency there will be for your joints to stiffen up.

Another quite pleasant form of exercise, although it might not seem to be exercise, is gardening. An afternoon spent in the back yard planting and cultivating flowers or vegetables is quite a vigorous way to pass the day. You derive much valuable movement from the constant and rhythmic bending of your hands and elbows, as well as the bending of your knees. It may seem difficult at first, particularly if your legs are the arthritically afflicted joints, because most gardening we have ever done has been on our knees. However, with slight modifications, you will be easily able to partake of this enjoyable hobby.

First, you can spend some of the time squatting, with the main part of your weight resting on your feet and not on your knees, as it would if you assumed the normal gardening position. Oftentimes we find ourselves gardening alongside a shelter-wall. In these cases you should make use of it by leaning or sitting on it while you garden. Another idea is to carry with you a low stool to sit on while you dig. Naturally you are able to water the foliage and the lawn while standing up, so this part of gardening will be no problem. Again, I would like to stress that you don't overexert yourself at the beginning. Thirty minutes outdoors the first time is quite sufficient.

Golf has long been one of my favorite sports, just as it is one of the most popular leisure-time activities in America. As my wife often tells our friends, if I cannot be found at home or in the swimming pool, it is almost a sure-fire bet that I will be on the golf course. This is because I have always found so much peaceful pleasure in playing a round of golf, as well as so much good exercise.

For the arthritic, golf has several advantages. It gives you the chance to be in the daylight and fresh air without calling for too strenuous activity. Usually you play golf with other people, which is always a more enjoyable experience than working at a sport by yourself. Finally, the movements in golf are quite beneficial to the arthritic. A smooth and complete backswing and follow-through utilize the joints of the wrists, elbows, hips, and shoulders, and to a large extent, the knee joints. The movements are smooth and not jerky, and in this respect are valuable.

However, do not go out to the golf course for a rousing eighteen-hole game the first chance you get. This could, again, be dangerous. You need to work up slowly to this sort of all-day diversion. Begin perhaps with a half hour of practice shots. Most golf courses have an area reserved for people who want to practice their strokes. After your muscles and joints become accustomed to this sort of activity, then you can attempt a more strenuous, and longer, time on the golf course.

Bowling is another sport which I highly recommend. Although you do not get the added benefits of being outdoors, you still get much good exercise from it. Bowling has the advantage, too, of putting you into a very social situation. That is, in addition to the exercise, you find yourself among a team of other people, in a congenial atmosphere, and many times this leads to after-bowling celebrations which keep you up and about and out of the confines of your home. Also, the knee-flexion and elbow-flexion you must perform while bowling are invaluable, because they are smooth and liquid-like manipulations of your joints, never jerky.

All of these types of exercise can be beneficial to you in your new, more mobile life. However, the problem still remains that a person who has had to confine him or herself to the inactive indoor life, and who has developed a definite pattern of life, will need more than a newly-acquired ability to get going. I well understand that if you have learned to shy away from participation in sports, you need incentive to get back into the habit.

In many cases the mere aspect of an improved self-image can supply this incentive. Many of my friends begin to think of themselves as active people, and they enjoy this role so much that it becomes a self-fulfilling prophecy. But with others, and indeed with the majority of people, it takes more than this.

One way to develop these new habits is to join an organization where the social aspect of exercise is emphasized as much as the physical benefits. There are many such organizations in existence, each with different purposes and different activities. For example, Audubon groups abound in the United States. In these societies, people go on bird-spotting hikes and walks in the countryside, which is a delightful way to pass the time, and to get valuable exercise and fresh air. Usually these excursions are held on weekends. You should check your local chapter of the Audubon Society for information and schedules.

The major source of group work can be found in senior citizens' organizations in your area. There are many kinds, each with different goals and activities. There are senior-citizen groups with golf tournaments, swimming days, gardening competitions, and bowling teams. So whatever your interest, do check on the local groups and choose one from which you can benefit. Often these groups organize weekend excursions to outdoor areas for the purpose of explorations or picnics, and these activities are always enjoyable and seldom expensive.

If you should happen to live in a "leisure world" community for senior citizens, then these groups and their activities may be right at your doorstep. However, if you do not, you should contact your local senior-citizen group, usually through the city or county offices.

SUPPORT FROM OTHER ARTHRITIS SUFFERERS AND GROUP EXERCISE

A very important source of advice and support for arthritis sufferers is the companionship of other persons with the same condition. You can learn a great deal from others about how to behave yourself, and by talking freely with friends and acquaintances in a similar position, you can more effectively face other social and family situations with a sense of self-assurance.

It is amazing how helpful other people with arthritis can be in having a positive effect on the psychological condition of their friends. Since so many people have come to me for advice about their problems, I have found that it sometimes helps to introduce the more hesitant ones to others for moral support. It sometimes helps for people to get together and exercise in groups; this way they can mark their own progress in a shared activity, and at the same time derive encouragement from observing the improvement of others.

When Margaret, the wife of a close friend, approached me and asked me for advice because she had heard from Bill, her husband, about my program, I suggested that she get together with another gal, a neighbor of hers, more advanced in the program. The results were marvelous. She and Cheryl hit it off immediately. Aside from their arthritis, they found they had many other things in common. From exercising together daily, they have become close friends, often lunching together and dining out with their husbands.

As I implied, at first Margaret was a little hesitant, but when she realized the progress Cheryl had made, and was able, by doing many of the same exercises appropriate for Cheryl, to see similar progress in her own condition, she came and thanked me for helping her not only to relieve her pain and suffering but to make a new and delightful friend.

Since each person's program of exercise will vary, when friends exercise together they may not necessarily be involved in the same activity simultaneously, but the bonus of having someone there to talk to and the reassurance derived from being engaged in a common effort at self-improvement make it that much easier to succeed with a program that has shown itself to work for countless others.

There are a number of advantages to your having friends who are also engaged in my program. Aside from the shared satisfaction of facing a common problem, and the social possibilities that can arise out of such shared activities, as in the case of Margaret and Cheryl, there is also the advantage of being able to follow my diet with others. Preparing a special meal for one is not nearly so enjoyable as sharing a meal with someone else, and, if you are both on the same regime, there is no griping from others. In retirement communities, where many people live alone and many are afflicted with arthritis, the sharing of wholesome meals, geared to improving general health and thereby countering arthritis, can provide a boost to the spirits as well as to health.

Mattie, a woman I went to high school with, now lives in a retirement community in California, and we've kept in touch over the years. When she told me she had arthritis, and that many of her friends there were also afflicted, I proposed my exercise program and diet to her, and suggested that she might want to let her friends in on them as well. She told me a very moving story of how many of the older people, who had given up on themselves before embarking on my program, had made marked improvement through the use of the methods I taught her and how they now enjoyed communal meals, prepared together in their homes, based on my diet. She said that they all were enjoying greater freedom of movement, better general health, and the social benefits of the shared activity had resulted in a number of new friendships and a feeling of a group effort which had not existed before. She even told me that one friend had said to her "I wish I had arthritis, so I could be in on the fun."

Mattie and her friends are just one example of the possibilities that can come of a combined effort of a group of arthritis sufferers to help themselves and bring about a general sense of well-being through shared activity. Your local chapter of the Arthritis Foundation may even be able to help you find or form a club in your area.

CHAPTER SEVEN

WARMHEARTED ADVICE ON HEAT TREATMENTS AND MASSAGE

The goal of physical therapies of all kinds is to maintain and improve the range of the movements of your joints and to increase the strength of the muscles that control them. In more advanced cases of osteoarthritis and rheumatoid arthritis, it is often required that people be given physical therapy in the form of another person's actively manipulating their limbs and joints. However, provided this is not required in your individual case, and that you have followed my exercise program and are thus making gradual improvement, there are other less drastic forms of physical therapy which can help you on your road to recovery.

As discussed earlier, heat treatments can relieve pain and restore mobility for short periods of time. While heat treatments by no means break, by themselves, the vicious circle inherent in an arthritic's lifestyle, as an adjunct to the exercise program they can be quite valuable. The application of heat in various forms is the commonest treatment used to combat pain and stiffness of arthritis. There are several sources of heat; among them are radiant, electric, and ultrasonic.

Radiant energy refers to rays of heat with wave lengths in the electromagnetic spectrum between the far infrared energy band on one side and the far ultraviolet area on the other. Between these two points we find the visible light spectrum, which is the source of luminous heat. Visible and infrared rays which are the sources of radiant heat, are different from the rays from other parts of this spectrum, because their action is primarily thermal. In other words, applying these kinds of rays usually means a heating sensation will accompany the application. Radiant energy, unlike sonic energy and X ray, has no deep biological action. This means that the only benefit you will get from radiant energy will occur because of the heat production.

There are two ways to transmit this heat to your body. One is called conduction and the other is convection. Conduction is by far the most preferred of the two. Conduction of radiant heat occurs when the energy, or warmth, is transferred by direct contact from the warm object to the cooler object. This form of treatment includes many "home type" treatments, such as hot water bottles, direct applications of heated bodies such as bricks, sandbags, irons, electric pads and blankets, and hot compresses. Conductive heating also includes more complicated and expensive, but not necessarily more effective, treatments such as fever cabinets, hot moist air, devices where hot water flows through various applications, and paraffin baths. Hot baths are also an example of a method of conductive heating.

On the other hand, convective heating is heating that is transmitted through the air or atmosphere to the body from a source not touching the body. This is infrared heat. The common form of this heat application is by luminous lamps. One device invented for this purpose is called the "baker." Bakers are heaters made up of several luminous bulbs which are backed by a reflector. Bakers are as effective as any other type of convective heating, and they are usually easily adjustable and quite portable, thus making them ideal for home use. Some radiant heat also is produced.

Heat treatments are as old as man himself, for a need to feel warm has always been identified with old people and arthritis. The reasons for this are obvious. Some people are particularly sensitive to the effects of cold, and their arthritis troubles are intensified by sitting in a draft. And how many times have you heard the older people in your family say that they could feel a storm coming on because of cold and dampness, the slight change in the weather, had already gotten into their bones? These are not frivolous claims. Nor is the nightly requirement of a hot water bottle, thick clothing, or an electric heating pad a crotchety idiosyncrasy of an older person. Heat has always been a recognized form of therapy, and warmth applied to aching joints is well known for providing relief. The simplest way to apply a heat treatment is certainly by using a hot water bottle. If this is used, remember never to fill it with water which is too hot and which causes pain. There is no advantage to extremely hot water in a treatment of this sort.

Many physical therapists use a heat treatment called a hydrocollator pack, which is a canvas bag filled with silica gel. The silica gel is able to hold the heat for a period of about twenty minutes after it has been heated in a hot water bath. In applying this treatment, the patient's skin is first covered with thick turkish towels, after which the hydrocollator pack is laid on. It is possible for a person to learn how to apply this sort of heat treatment to himself, and it has been found by hospitals to be much more successful than the hot water bottle. It can be purchased for about five dollars a pack in hospital supply stores.

It is important to note that this sort of treatment is an example of moist heat, which is the kind of heat that should normally be used therapeutically. The use of moist heat creates an efficient coupling agent to conduct the heat onto the tissues. There are other forms of dry heat which from time to time may be utilized, such as heat lamps and infrared heat, but generally osteoarthritics derive more relief from moist heat than from dry heat.

If however, dry heat is used, it should only be in the form of mild infrared radiation. It may be given for fifteen to thirty minutes several times a day. The maximum heat which can comfortably be tolerated should be focused on the painful joint. The infrared lamp should be placed from two to three feet from your body, depending on the reflector and the sensitivity of the areas of your body which are being treated. The main thing in using dry heat is that you avoid skin burn. Having to take this precaution is why dry heat does not relieve as much as moist heat. With moist heat, the moisture acts as a conductor, and brings the heat deep inside your limbs. With dry heat there is no such conductor, and the heat from the lamp tends to burn the surface instead of penetrating deep into the afflicted parts of your body. One way to avoid skin burn is to place a towel over the afflicted area. The towel does not interfere with penetration and it acts as a conductor, sometimes taking the role of moisture in moist heat (only not as effectively), thus helping to prevent skin burn. Infrared rays penetrate about half an inch into the tissues of your skin.

The simplest type of heat lamp is a cup-shaped, polished reflector. These usually come with a clamp, so that they can be attached to whatever is at hand. Any electrical outlet will support this kind of lamp, and you can pick them up most anywhere for no more than five dollars.

The one advantage of dry heat of this kind is that, unlike hot compresses, it never cools down. You can, technically, leave it focused on your arthritic joints for much longer periods of time. However, this is only a superficial advantage. A compress will usually last about twenty minutes, and this is quite long enough for any application at any one time. It is much better to have several shorter applications spaced out over a long period of time, the course of a day for example, than to fatigue and overload the afflicted joint by one quite long application. So, in the end, I see no distinct advantage for the use of dry heat over moist heat.

Besides the above-mentioned hydrocollator packs there are other types of moist heat treatments, some of which are easier to use at home by the arthritic himself.

Hot packs can be applied much in the same way as the hot water bottle. First, you should tear an old blanket or sheet into strips, approximately one to one-and-a-half feet square. Very heavy towels or old wool cloth can also be used. Dip them into very hot water that is about 115° F. When you have done this and have made sure they are soaked through, wring them out carefully and wrap them about the afflicted joint. Several layers of hot towels should be placed around the joint, and they should extend well above and below the joint. Once the wrapping is completed, take a piece of plastic or oiled silk, or even heavy waxed paper, and enclose the entire area in this. This is to keep the moisture and warmth from escaping. You can also wrap several hot water bottles or an electric heating pad around the area, finally enclosing the entire treatment in a large, warmed blanket. Leave the equipment in place for twenty to forty minutes. This treatment can be applied two to three times daily. With this treatment you can work on several joints at a time. This is especially effective for acutely painful or swollen joints.

Of course for everyday and all-day use, one of the simplest techniques of heat application is merely the wearing of a warm piece of clothing, always over the afflicted area. This method is age-old, and is well known among hardworking peasants all over the world who do back-breaking work. In Poland, the men often wear rabbit skins covering their backs when they go out hunting or to work in the fields. In southern France and throughout Spain and Italy the people wear the wide belt-like, cinched cummerbunds which are knitted from thick, warm wool. As a matter of fact, these are so widely worn that they are very much a part of the national peasant costume. In England, for hundreds of years, a cloth known as Doll's flannel has been applied traditionally to an aching back. It is from this that thermal underwear developed.

Today, many osteoarthritics can be greatly helped simply by our heeding these generations of tried and true wisdom. An elastic bandage around the knee, as an example, provides much relief when worn under clothing (provided, of course, it is not too tight) for the warmth it supplies rather than for any support it may or may not give.

Another common treatment for an aching joint is a "mustard plaster" or other liniment application. A variety of chemicals included in these liniments interreact to provide valuable warmth after the application is on the skin. This is the effect of "heat rubs" and other such commercial products.

A last quite effective heat treatment, especially suitable for arthritic hands, is the application of hot wax, or the paraffin treatment. The advantage of the paraffin treatment is that, unlike a hot pack, it can bring heat to all sides of the joints of the fingers and the hands. The paraffin treatment can be referred to as a "wax bath."

A particular kind of paraffin wax is used for this method, and it is important to use only this kind (it can be obtained from most any pharmacist), because most other waxes melt at quite high temperatures, while this one melts at a lower temperature. If another wax were used, when you dipped your hands in you would burn them quite badly.

Another very important point is that you must never melt this wax directly on an electric or a gas stove, because the wax catches fire easily. You must melt it in a double boiler. This causes it to be gently steamed from underneath, and this way it is only heated to the temperature that is required to melt it. After it is melted, you must let it cool a bit until a "skin" is formed on the top of it. At this point you can proceed with the dipping.

After you have purchased the wax, separate three or four pounds of paraffin from the main bulk of the wax, and warm it in the top of an ordinary kitchen double boiler to 190° F. When it melts entirely, you should remove it from the heat and allow it to cool until it drops to approximately 120° F. You can gauge the temperature of the heat by using a simple candy thermometer, and it is essential that you be able to tell exactly when it reaches these temperatures. Otherwise, you might severely burn your hands. At 120° F., a thin film of solidified wax, the "skin" I mentioned before, should cover the surface of the heated wax.

Next, it is time to dip your hands. Dip them one at a time. Each should be dipped in and out of the melted wax four or five times. After each immersion you should allow the wax to dry a bit, so at the next immersion a layered effect will build up over your hands. After approximately five separate immersions of each hand, a thick coating of wax should be built up on your hands. At this point you should wrap both your hands in oiled silk, oilcloth, or thin sheets of plastic. This should be covered in a light blanket.

You can leave the wrappings on your hands for twenty to thirty minutes. After that time, remove the covers and then strip the wax away gently from your skin. The wax can be returned to a receptacle for future remelting.

This, by the way, is an excellent time to practice your exercises. At this time your joints are warm and elastic, and usually the paraffin treatment will relieve much of the pain and inflammation, making self-manipulation possible.

Another very effective form of physical therapy is that of massage. Again though, it is merely a temporary measure. It lends much relief to aching joints for short periods of time, and as an adjunct to the basic exercise program, it can be quite beneficial. However, used on its own, massage only lends relief for a matter of minutes, and does little to restore mobility to stiff and aching joints.

The benefits of massage are readily understood. It is always soothing and relaxing to receive a gentle massage on your tense neck and shoulder muscles after a frantic day at work. In the same way, when an arthritic is in severe pain, his muscles become very tense and rigid. This naturally increases any discomfort he might already be feeling in his joints. A person who is adept at massage can relax the muscles, thereby relieving much of the pain temporarily. This, however, does not solve the problem of arthritis.

Massage is usually considered to be the most familiar and most pleasant form of treatment of arthritic pain. It has been used for centuries, for as long as man has tried to treat muscle and joint disorders. Arthritic massage, however, is a precarious technique, and should only be attempted by a trained physical therapist. Do not allow anyone else to try to massage your body, for great harm can result.

Massage is usually done at home by a physical therapist, or at one of the many clinics throughout the country which specialize in this occupation. There are many home-visiting organizations which have a retinue of physical therapists who are happy to make house calls for people who might otherwise not receive the benefits of this treatment. These services are usually obtainable by calling your county or city health department. Also, arthritis clinics exist as adjuncts of many hospitals, and one can find qualified physical therapists at these places, who have been trained in the massage of arthritic joints. I would like to emphasize that it is imperative to allow only a trained therapist to work on your body in this fashion. Mis-manipulation, particularly of the back and spinal region, could very well cause permanent damage.

Massage consists of repeated pressures upon the skin with

the side or the flat of the hand. It is done quite gently at first, occasionally intensifying a bit later on. Gentle stroking causes muscle relaxation, while more intense and quicker stroking causes muscle contraction. Both techniques may be used.

I would like to point out that arthritic massage is normally applied only to the muscles in the region surrounding the inflamed joints. This is quite important, because massage of the joints themselves could easily cause your condition to worsen. Yet when the muscles *around* the joints are massaged, the tension is relaxed in the entire area, thus relieving much of the pain of the afflicted joints. You see, massage causes increased blood flow in the muscles. In certain types of arthritis, the blood vessels contract, blocking the normal amount of blood from flowing into the arthritic area. When the muscles are massaged, the vessels enlarge or dilate, relieving the problem to a certain extent. Muscle tone is often improved with regular massage, too.

A normal massage period varies in duration according to the number of joints which are afflicted, the size of the surface, and the intensity of affliction. However, to give you some idea, a normal, all-over body massage lasts approximately one hour, so the individual arthritic joint massage would obviously be shorter. Generally, it can be expected that the average time for an arm massage is from five to ten minutes; a leg massage, ten to fifteen minutes; and approximately fifteen minutes for a back massage. The therapist will usually begin the session with very light stroking. In these periods, the hands are passed gently over the skin in circular motions. The movements are always smooth and rhythmical, and at this point quite slow, so as not to exceed fifteen strokes per minute. A good therapist can sense how much pressure to apply, and when to begin applying the pressure. This knowledge and ability, however, come from much practice and experience with the art of massage. Later on, other movements emphasized are various degrees of stroking, the most pressurized being referred to as "deep stroking." Also used are various forms of compression, including kneading and friction, percussion (which refers to various degrees of slapping, tapping, or gentle beating), and finally vibration. All of these methods may be utilized, as long as none of them is addressed to the joint area directly.

It is usually advised when your joints are acutely painful— that is, if they are inflamed—that you refrain from massage until the pain and inflammation subside. It can only be harmful to manipulate further already painful areas. As the swelling and redness begin to disappear one can begin to massage the areas using only gentle and deep stroking motions. This should be performed for about ten minutes, twice a day. Also, it is good to massage these painful joints only after a heat application. At this time, the afflicted areas are most elastic, and consequently, most receptive to manipulation.

Usually during a massage the room is kept at 70° F. or more. This is very important in creating the best possible environment for your body. Only the part of your body that is being massaged is exposed.

There are several other more complicated kinds of massage which have proven to be quite beneficial. Some physical therapists prefer to apply an ointment or a liniment while they massage painful limbs. There are several kinds on the market with many different purposes. Many have chemicals that react on your body to create heat, which creates a better environment for the massage. Others, when rubbed into the skin, open up the blood vessels of the skin, causing an increased blood supply, which oftentimes helps in relieving pains. Traditional liniment compounds include mustard, camphor, and various oils. Most can be easily purchased from drugstores, but usually the physical therapist will have a preference and will carry his own liniment or ointment with him.

All of these methods of physical therapy are valuable as adjuncts to your basic exercise program, for, as we have seen earlier, the less pain you are in, the more you will want to move around. The more you want to move, the less stiffness will occur, and consequently, the less pain when you do move. This is the nature of the vicious circle which the arthritic lives in, and anything we can do to end that circle is certainly to be advised. However, it must be remembered that these treatments are only temporary, and the only way I have ever seen to rid a person more permanently of the pain of arthritis is through the basic exercise program which I described earlier.

CHAPTER EIGHT

SEX AND THE OSTEOARTHRITIC

Here we arrive at what is doubtless a delicate subject, yet what is also a very important one to all who suffer from arthritis. We are all aware of the strain the sexual frustration during illness puts on our lives and our relationships with our loved ones. To live with arthritis, a permanent illness, indeed magnifies that particular frustration immensely. It is obvious to almost everyone that a healthy sex life is essential to the mental health of married couples. Those couples where one or both partners develop arthritis certainly have an added strain put on them.

A very important question to be discussed here is that of a definition of a normal, healthy sex life. What exactly is this? The frequency and the kind of sex would be factors to consider when discussing this, yet these factors are entirely dependent on individual preferences. There exists an incredibly wide range in attitudes among men and women toward sex. Even within families, there exists a wide range of opinions. What this points toward is that there is no absolute upon which the normalcy of a couple's sexual life can be judged. The frequency of intercourse, the time of day, and the circumstances of intercourse all are purely matters of choice and pleasure.

Many couples who are happy make love twice a day, many once a month or less. Some couples have intercourse in the morning, some at night in the dark. Just as frequency varies widely, so does the amount and kind of foreplay. Some people enjoy a period of complicated sex-play and ritual before they actually make love; others find this unnecessary. All these things are solely up to the discretion of the individuals, and no one can say what is proper or healthy as regards a normal sex life. What is normal to one couple, may be either excessive or minimal to another.

The final judgment, then, should be passed only by the couple. Consequently, when one or both members are dissatisfied with their sex life, it is time to take a meaningful and close look at it. It is here that problems may arise, from the discontent of one or both of the parties. Among arthritics, this is frequently a large and common concern. However, a very important factor to be considered is that very seldom does osteoarthritis biologically interfere with a couple's sex life. By this I mean that except in cases where hip deformity is extremely great (and I will discuss that occurrence later), the interference that osteoarthritis causes is purely an exterior and/or mental one.

The exterior interference is, of course, caused when joints are so painful that the individual cannot move easily, let alone participate in a vigorous period of sexual activity. This will usually occur among people who are afflicted in their legs and/or backs. In these cases, a high level of mutual understanding is necessary, for the pain may not subside after one night, but may continue for several nights, even for weeks. This is understood to be quite frustrating to *both* parties involved. Intimate conversations and airing of frustrations is strongly advised, as well as a large dose of patience. For however much talk goes on (and I hope it will be enough to keep the communication channels open), the physical frustration will still remain until the pain has subsided enough so that the sexual urges can be fulfilled. The only thing I know of which can truly cope with this frustration is lots of love and patience.

There are no easy answers to these external roadblocks. When a person's joints give him this much pain, sexual participation is simply an impossibility. However, there are several methods of relaxation which might be utilized to help the pain and inflammation subside so the individual will more rapidly be able to resume his role in the relationship and participate in the sexual experience once more.

Obviously, the less pain you are feeling, the more you will want to participate in a sexual experience, and the better will be that experience, both for you and for your mate. Consequently, it is advisable to prepare yourself for sexual intercourse with heat treatments to the afflicted joints. It is directly following such treatments that your body will be the most pliable and given to sexual activity. Mild massage is also recommended directly preceding sexual intercourse.

It is best not to attempt to have intercourse when your joints are at their stiffest, which usually means the period of time after a long day of hard work. You most likely are fatigued or in pain when you come home from work, and to try to make love at this point would probably compound frustration upon a long day of frustration.

Another important modification you can make to encourage sexual fulfillment is to raise the temperature of your home by setting the thermostat a few degrees higher. This technique acts in much the same way as it does when you are being given a massage. In that case, the warmer temperature of the room acts as a muscle relaxant, making your muscles more pliable so the therapist will be able to achieve full rotational capacity with your joints and muscles. In a sexual situation, the higher temperature of the room serves to relax your muscles in just the same way, thereby eliminating some of the pain and allowing you to concentrate more on sexual arousal.

Generally, the various localized methods of relieving arthritic pain which we have discussed in previous chapters can all be modified and used to great advantage in sexual situations to eliminate pain from the joint areas.

Oftentimes one of the main problems in this area is lack of creativity. The most frequently used sexual position of the woman lying on her back with the man on top of her is not always the least painful for arthritic joints. The woman with arthritis in any part of her legs, *i.e*, her hips, knees or ankles, can experience great amounts of pain when attempting to part her legs wide enough to achieve full satisfaction. Pressure is often applied on just the most painful joints in this position. The male arthritic, in this position, also probably experiences much pain. In the first place there is a great deal of physical exertion required of him in the pelvic area, which, if he has arthritis in his hips or legs, will greatly irritate and might even injure these joints. If his arthritis is in his back, the constant bending and twisting of the spine is bound to be quite painful. If the arthritis lies in his arms, shoulders, or wrists, he cannot possibly use these limbs for support or leverage in the sexual act without incurring a great deal of pain.

Obviously, then, it is wise to seek out other positions for intercourse. It may be more beneficial for the man to be on his back with the woman on top, or for the man to sit in a chair while the woman lowers herself, gently, onto him. There exist many positions which can and definitely should be tried, until you settle on those that cause you the least pain. There are hundreds of sexual manuals to which you can refer as guides or for suggestions.*

*Extreme hip deformity creates a severe block to sexual intercourse. It makes normal intercourse impossible. Fortunately, many advances have been made in the area of hip surgery, which relieve the deformity and make sex possible again. If this is your particular problem, you should check with the arthritis clinic at your local hospital as to the possibilities of this surgery. Without this surgery, one still should not give up. As I have said, there are hundreds of positions which can be utilized while making love, and simply because the most common ones are no longer possible there is no reason to give up entirely.

Let me emphasize the importance of this kind of experimentation. I realize that with many people, even those who have been married a long time, it is very much a taboo subject. Yet I believe it is more important to learn to discuss these matters freely if you find that arthritic pain is causing you much sexual frustration. And please, be the *first* to bring the subject up between you and your mate. Don't wait for your partner to skirt the issue. *If you do, neither of you may ever get the courage to discuss it,* and you may spend years in sexually frustrating circumstances. Take the matter in hand and take the risk yourself, for what you can gain from doing so far outvalues whatever decorum you may be trying to preserve.

The other interference, as I mentioned earlier, that osteoarthritis causes in a person's sexual fulfillment is psychological.

Arousal is very much a psychological process, regardless of the physical effects we may see in it. All sorts of psychological stimuli go into the physical arousal of a person. In a man, the signs of arousal are obvious; they are less obvious in a woman, but of course just as important. Consequently, once you have conquered the external problems mentioned above, if you are still having troubles they undoubtedly are psychological, and most likely have to do with arousal problems.

There are many mutual practices which can be engaged in to aid the achievement of arousal. One of the partners might learn a bit of gentle and uncomplicated massage from the physical therapist. This could then be performed very gently prior to love-making. Another possibility is a mutual warm bath. This has been quite effective when employed immediately preceding sexual intercourse. It relaxes both parties, soothes the joints of the one who is afflicted, and also acts as a medium of arousal. I recommend this highly.

As an osteoarthritic, you may feel separated from the mainstream of society merely by the fact that you have sexual problems of this kind. You may feel that your disease has incapacitated you, or that you are different from most people. Past the external problems, this is simply not true. Interestingly enough, ninety percent of the sexual problems which occur within couples where one partner, or both, have arthritis are *exactly the same problems that effect non-arthritics.* Remember this, for it is important in overcoming many of your psychological misgivings. You are no different sexually from anyone else. The problems are the age-old, typical problems that sexual counsellors deal with every day. Despite their immediate and serious nature, they are therefore normal problems. Being an arthritic *in no way* means that your sexual life is doomed to failure, or even that it will be particularly difficult, once you have gotten around the pain.

When I was working and living in southern California, I met a man in West Los Angeles who ran a pet shop near where I lived. My wife and I bought our collie from Scott, and often had occasion to frequent his pet store for supplies and advice. Over the course of several years, he became one of my closest friends. A couple of years ago Scott became badly afflicted with arthritis, and he had to stop working in the store. His wife took over the business, and it was her cheery face that I began to see behind the counter every day. By this time, though, Scott's family and my family lived in the same part of town, and I used to drop by his house whenever I could to see how he was doing.

The minute I had discovered that he had arthritis, I suggested he work out a plan of exercise. Since he spent so much time at home, he was able to begin a serious and concentrated effort at these exercises, and in no time at all he had regained enough mobility and had lost enough pain so that he could get around his home. He soon reached the point where he could even putter around in the garden some. However, he still could not spend the day on his feet without incurring a great deal of pain, and so his wife continued running the family business. What had happened here was a complete role-reversal. Scott had taken over the duties of a housewife, while his wife had assumed those of her husband. While this sort of role-reversal doesn't bother some people, and in fact is quite common in Sweden, it very much bothered Scott. He had spent many years as the breadwinner in his family and his identity and self-pride were very much tied up with this role.

I was visiting him one afternoon when he became quite agitated and explained very nervously to me that he and his wife had been having sexual problems, which he attributed to something he thought his arthritis was doing to him biologically. Knowing I had had some experience with arthritic people, he thought perhaps I knew of a drug which could counteract the effects he thought he was having.

After much more probing and conversation, I did indeed have an answer, although it was not at all the answer that Scott was expecting. I patiently explained to him that arthritis has no known biological effect on one's sexuality. What I believed was happening was his loss of self-esteem, and this was affecting his potency as a sexual partner. Clearly, Scott no longer saw himself as a "man," and this bothered him intensely.

We talked about this feeling quite a bit, and he admitted that this was quite true, and that it might even be the cause of his impotency. I suggested that he open communications with his wife much more, and that he might even consider seeing a marriage counsellor who specialized in sexual problems.

Scott out-and-out refused to do this, but he did agree to discuss his problems with his wife more freely. I also suggested that he try to spend a certain amount of time each day at the pet store—certainly not long enough to harm him physically, but short of that—a couple of hours which would not be too strenuous. As it turned out, his wife had been needing his help for several months, but she didn't want to bother him with business problems, so she hadn't said anything. Scott began to spend three hours a day at the shop, for the most part doing work on the books. This gave his wife more time to spend on the actual running of the shop. Of prime importance, he began to feel more self-esteem because he was assuming responsibilities for the well-being of the family, which he had previously relinquished.

Scott's arthritis has improved so much over the last months as a result of his exercise program and his dedication that he and his wife now share the responsibilities of the pet shop completely. The last time I spoke with him he seemed to be a happy, robust person again, and he mentioned that his sexual problems had long ago been solved.

What this points to is that Scott's problem was the age-old one of a man *feeling that he had been emasculated*. This is a serious problem, of course, and a bit more understanding and communication may be required of a couple in which one or both of the partners are arthritic, than by an otherwise normal couple. The arthritic couple will need to make adjustments in their lives. Yet this required extra communication can also work as an advantage. Because you are forced to keep healthy communication open, and because you are forced to have a bit more patience with each other, you tend to develop a deeper relationship.

These self-esteem problems are not peculiar to the male in a relationship. Often it is the woman who is afflicted by arthritis, and who develops arousal problems with regard to sex. For the woman a psychological part of sexuality may be in her looking and feeling attractive. If a woman feels attractive, she will be, and will be more given to participating in sexual intercourse. If, on the other hand, a woman feels that her husband and her family, not to mention all her friends, find her unattractive, she usually will act according to that belief, and will not feel sexually alluring.

Unfortunately, many times arthritis sets in just at the time when a woman starts to age, biologically. The two occurrences cannot be linked to each other except coincidentally. However, when a woman begins to go through menopause, she undergoes a dramatic psychological change which is very difficult for a man to understand. During this change, she may begin to deeply question her femininity, or become unsure of herself. If menopause is then accompanied with the onset of arthritis, this can create a very trying time, indeed, for the woman. She is already growing older and does not feel as attractive as she used to. Finally, if she becomes afflicted with arthritis and experiences extreme pain during sexual intercourse, her self-doubts are compounded.

This obviously is a time which calls for immense understanding and patience on the part of her mate. (Statistically, the divorce rate is quite high during this period in a woman's life.) Several techniques can be adopted. A more-often-than-usual affirmation of your love for your wife is never out of place. Neither are scattered compliments about her appearance. These things will serve to boost her sense of self-esteem. A bunch of flowers or a box of candy will do wonders.

Another problem is that many times a woman who is becoming increasingly afflicted with arthritis finds it difficult to take care of her appearance. She is in just too much pain to get out of the house. Anything that increases self-respect is important to explore. If the woman cannot leave her home, it is vital to make available to her all manner of appearance-modifiers—cosmetics, hair styles, clothing, etc. *Great effort should be made* to bring these items and possibilities to her. What is even better than this, though, is making special arrangements to transport the woman to places where these items are available. Just getting out of the house will be of invaluable therapeutic value because women who are undergoing this difficult period particularly tend to want to hide at home. This practice only encourages the disadvantages of the illness instead of trying to overcome them.

Another difficulty in this stage of both a woman's and a man's life is that they tend to lose all interest in hobbies. This oftentimes is out of necessity. Knitting may become impossible when a woman is afflicted with arthritis. Gardening, woodcarving, and other once-enjoyed activities may become at best quite painful and difficult. Yet these sorts of pastimes add to a person's self-esteem, and it is quite important to help the person find new ones to replace the old ones. Always remember that any element of the person's life which adds to his or her self-esteem, aids the person in feeling a sexual identity again.

I would like to express some final words about a practice which many couples resort to. That is the acquisition of single beds. Usually this occurs when one partner is going through a particularly painful arthritic period. The other partner, out of consideration, generally, decides it would be less frustrating to move to a separate bed and sometimes even to a separate room. This is to allow the afflicted partner peace and quiet while sleeping, as he usually has difficulty enough with all the pain from his arthritis.

This separation is not always the wisest course available. Often the arthritic partner may feel rejected and abnormal. Sleeping apart may lead to intense psychological feelings of rejection and separation for both partners, which can only be destructive to the relationship.

An essential part of married life is being able to lie together in bed, to end each day in close proximity to the loved one. Good communication is often based on the ability to talk to one another in bed, to touch each other, and generally to lie together. That closeness can be invaluable in keeping healthy lines of caring and communication open. So I would advise thinking cautiously about this sort of move before you undertake it.

There are several good pamphlets presently in publication which can help you in developing new attitudes toward sexuality. If you would like further advice on this subject, I would suggest that you write to the Arthritis and Rheumatism Council, at 8–10 Charing Cross Road, London, WC2H OHN, England, for any information they might have, and in particular, for the pamphlet entitled, "Marriage, Sex, and Arthritis." In addition you might contact the Arthritis Foundation, Inc., 3400 Peachtree Road, N.E., Atlanta, Ga. 30326.

CHAPTER NINE

DRUGS AND DIETS

DRUGS

If you have been afflicted with arthritis for any period of time at all I am sure you have experienced the disappointments of the many pain relievers. Time and again arthritics are encouraged to become excited about new forms of medication that are on the market, and time and again they are disappointed in the results, for it remains a basic fact that any drug you put into your system that is strong enough to smother a disease like arthritis, or to stop the pain of this disease on a long-term basis, *will inevitably make other changes in your body*, some of them not so welcome. So, either the drugs are not strong enough to do any good, in which case they have no effect on any part of your body, or they are so strong that while curbing the symptoms of arthritis, they also wreak havoc on other parts of your body. This is a sad, sad truth that more arthritics each day are discovering.

There is a very basic fact involved here. Anything you put into your body, including food, water, coffee, cigarette smoke, alcohol, or any of the wide range of prescription and non-prescription drugs, alters your body chemistry in some way. It is the case that some short-term uses of certain elements will not alter your body permanently. Obviously, a cup of coffee, though the caffeine in it will make you "hyper" for a few hours, will not permanently or drastically change your metabolism. Some substances, of course, change your body for the better. A piece of fruit for dessert instead of a piece of cake would certainly have a more healthy effect on your body. Vitamins, taken in moderation, are good for your body. So it is all-important to try to minimize the amounts of substances we ingest which harm our bodies, and to try to maximize those that create good effects. It is important here to note that some seemingly beneficial drugs have overpoweringly bad effects which completely outweigh their good effects. You must carefully decide for yourself, with the aid of your doctor, where your priorities lie.

For example, I have seen aspirin, as simple a compound as it might seem, have bad effects on people. I knew a taxi driver in Hollywood who used to work around the studio quite a bit. In those days I did not have any understanding of the arthritis problem, but I remember that he used to get pains and stiffness quite badly in his neck and back, and that for long periods at a time he wasn't able to drive a cab. He explained to me one day that he had had arthritis for several years, and that over this period he had tried many different kinds of medication. At one time his doctor prescribed massive doses of aspirin, which certainly relieved the pain, but the burning effect of the aspirin on his stomach became too much for him. The aspirin ate out a hole in his stomach, and gave him what seemed to be an ulcer. At any rate, the symptoms were the same, and even after he had stopped taking the aspirin he still had to nurse his "ulcer." In this case, the medication was injurious to him, and it was not worth it to him to continue taking it. Unfortunately, he was left with two problems in the end: arthritis *and* a damaged stomach lining.

So it is advisable to be careful with all medications, including those, like aspirin, which seem to be the least harmful. Aspirin may not have this effect on your system, but there is the possibility that it might. Certainly it is inadvisable to experiment with any medication, whether prescription or non-prescription, without the advice of your doctor. Throughout the following discussion of some of the many drugs available it is important to remember that they act only as temporary pain or symptom relievers. The only permanent way I have found to modify arthritis and to eliminate much of the pain is through a comprehensive exercise program such as I have described in this book. Drugs are only an adjunct to exercise. Drugs will not bring you increased mobility in your joints. Although they are able to modify the pain for short periods of time, it still remains that once their effects have worn off, the symptoms of your disease will return.

Aspirin and other salicylates are perhaps the most common drugs used in treating osteoarthritis. Salicylates include Bufferin and sodium salicylate. However, as with aspirin, small doses are prescribed in order to avoid any side effects. For controlling pain in particularly inflamed periods, many people find small doses of these drugs helpful. A usual perscription might be two tablets four times daily after meals and at bedtime. But I would like to stress that these are only temporary measures. Long-term ingestion of these drugs could radically alter your body chemistry. People with bronchial asthma, or those people who already have ulcers of the stomach or small intestine should indulge in the use of salicylates moderately, and then only under supervision of their doctors.

Another problem with these kinds of drugs is that to be effective, the dose taken is often quite near the level producing toxic symptoms. There is a fine line between effectiveness and toxicity, and consequently one should never self-prescribe this, or any other, medication for arthritis. Toxic symptoms include nausea and ringing in the ears.

Note should be taken that there are hundreds of patent drugs that are advertised widely in all the media which contain aspirin, aspirin-like drugs, or aspirin derivatives. Many of these tout monumental results in relieving pain, but no patent medicine will work better than plain aspirin, for they all base their pain-killing effects on the aspirin they contain. Just as the advantages are the same (not to mention a good bit more expensive) in these drugs, so the disadvantages are the same. There is no patent drug on the market which has overcome the problems that aspirin encounters.

Codeine has been prescribed frequently in past years for sufferers of severe joint pain from arthritis. However, it must be remembered that codeine is a narcotic. If it is used on a long-term or regular basis, the user can become addicted to it. Since arthritis is a chronic disease, it is unwise to get into the habit of using codeine to kill pain, even intermittently. And certainly, use of this or similar drugs should only be undertaken under strict medical supervision.

Sedatives are another class of drugs which are occasionally prescribed in arthritis. This is because the pain, and the frustration which results from stiffness, often cause nervousness. Sleeplessness also becomes a problem when the individual is in too much pain to fall asleep at night. Phenobarbital has been found to be quite effective. Also used are several newer drugs such as Thorazine, Miltown, and various sleeping pills. Again, these should never be used on a regular basis, for the harmful effects they can have on your body far outweigh any advantages they might bring.

A great amount of controversy still rages about the subject of steroid hormones. These are hormones which have been synthetically composed. They usually offer prompt relief from arthritic symptoms. These drugs include many types: ACTH, hydrocortisone, cortisone, prednisone, prednisolone, and triamcinolone. These are all closely related in that they have much the same effect on the body. They combat inflammation.

At first when these compounds were discovered they were believed to be cures for various kinds of arthritis. Unfortunately, as time progressed and experimentation results came in, it was found that these drugs were simply another form of symptom suppressant. The basic progress of the disease continues with the use of these drugs, even though while under their influence the patient certainly experiences a vanishing of pain and inflammation. Yet immediately after ceasing to take these drugs the symptoms return in full force.

There are several problems that have developed as side effects of these drugs, and this is the cause of all the controversy. A sufficiently long experimentation period has not been available with steroids to be able to prove their advantages or to control their disadvantages. The major problem is that in large enough doses to be effective, the drugs alter the internal secretions of various glands, making it necessary to stop the medication. Much experimentation is being carried on today in an attempt to overcome this problem. One quite successful solution is to administer small doses several times a day or to take one larger dose around 4:00 P.M. when the glands are at their lowest working level. An interesting and more positive use of these hormones is that of temporarily suppressing pain and swelling to allow a complete program of physical therapy, rest, and exercise to take place unhindered. In other words, the hormones temporarily stave off the symptoms while the individual employs more basic and long-reaching methods. Thus, after a few weeks or months, the hormones are stopped and the patient has gained from their use. But it should be noted that it is an indirect gain. Steroid hormones are in no way a cure for arthritis.

Unfortunately, the steroid hormones have quite a dramatic effect which is overly encouraging. Hydrocortisone needs particular examination here. Often it is injected into a particularly painful joint. It has considerable effect when used locally in this way. When a joint is especially inflamed, hydrocortisone often brings about symptomatic remission, including relief from pain, reduced swelling, and heat in the involved area.

But it is the same problem as with all other medications which we have discussed: A dose large enough to have an effect will alter the body in a harmful way, yet a dose small enough to avoid this alteration will have little or no effect on the disease. Steroid hormones produce indigestion and stomach ulcers. They also have frequently been known to weaken the bones and muscles. If large doses are used, after a few months of treatment people's faces grow to be quite rounded and red, a condition which is known as "moon face." Another side effect is that many women tend to grow facial hair, and a large hump on the nape of the neck.

Any individual who is being given steroid hormones is required to carry with him at all times a card which identifies him as a steroid user. The reason for this is that drastic complications will occur if use of steroids is stopped suddenly. Consequently, the card is a record of the individual's personal steroid prescription, including how much he or she takes and for how long it's been taken, as well as the prescribing physician's name, address, and telephone number. In case of accident, the attending physician will be able, then, to continue the essential administration of the steroids. This requirement demonstrates the severity of these drugs.

Also used to combat arthritis are massive doses of different vitamins, including Vitamin D and Vitamin B_{12}. This technique has gained immense popularity lately but it has not had proper experimentation or research. I feel that this sort of fad therapy is quite dangerous and its advantages are totally unproven. Even if there were validated good results, *which (so far) there are not*, it probably would be the same old case which we have seen again and again. That is, to take enough of these vitamins to do any good borders on the toxic level, which causes unwanted effects on the body. And to take so little that these effects are avoided means that the vitamins will do no particular good for your body or your arthritis.

DIET

Diet is all-important in the control of arthritis, but I must first emphasize how that is true. It is often thought that certain foods will cause the remission of arthritis or its symptoms, and so ingestion of these is often recommended. This could not be further from the truth. Eating large amounts of oils or green vegetables, or any of the other fad foods which frequently come into popularity, is only unhealthy and dangerous, and has absolutely no effect on arthritis. I want to emphasize that to this day no cure has been discovered for arthritis. It is a chronic disease. The only possible solution is treatment of the symptoms, and the only long-term effective treatment of this kind which I have found is that of exercise and a healthier way of life.

And yet *diet does indeed figure very importantly in your new way of life as an active arthritic.* This is because degenerative joint disease, or osteoarthritis, is in fact a breakdown of the joints of the body. One of the main causes of this breakdown is undue stress put on the joints. Just as we have seen that taking pressure off the joints relieves pain, so it is true that taking this pressure off in a more permanent way slows down the process of degeneration. Any time a joint is forced to shift excess amounts of weight, it is doing more than its share, more than the purpose for which it exists. Our joints cannot stand to support great amounts of weight disproportionate to the size of the joints. Consequently, if we are overweight, even five or ten pounds, we are helping along the inevitable degeneration of the joints.

It is very important not to carry around excess weight. This is where the role of proper diet comes in. When we maintain a proper weight our joints undergo less strain. Indeed, many people who suffer from osteoarthritis find that their symptoms disappear after they lose twenty or thirty pounds. This is because the weight alone was straining, and thus degenerating, their joints.

An actress I worked with many times experienced just such an occurrence. We played opposite each other several times when we were relatively young. At one meeting, we were to begin filming in a few weeks, but when we met to read through the script, she had, to the amazement of all, put on about thirty pounds. I had not seen her for two years, and I was very much surprised that she, an actress who must scrupulously watch her weight, would have let this happen.

Normally, the producers would have hired a new actress, but we all loved this one so dearly that we agreed to put off shooting while she lost some of the weight. When we left the conference room that afternoon, she confided in me that she also had gotten arthritis, and she hoped that it, too, wouldn't interfere with shooting. She said her back, as well as swelling in her knee joints, were giving her quite a bit of pain from time to time.

At this point in my life I knew nothing about arthritis or its causes; however, I did think it a bit peculiar that she would gain weight and begin to suffer from arthritis at the same time. Also, I was surprised about the arthritis because she was not even my age at the time—she was only thirty years old. I tried to reassure her, and urged her to go on a sensible diet.

The next time I saw her was for the beginning of filming a couple of months later. By this time she had lost nearly twenty-five pounds. She looked terrific again. Later I found that she felt terrific, too. Apparently her arthritis had disappeared gradually as she began to lose weight. To this day, nearly forty years later, she still maintains a healthy weight, and has never suffered again from the arthritis.

Extra weight becomes a problem with older people, just when we need most to control our weight. Many factors can account for this. People who have never had to watch their weight are no longer doing the same amount of exercise as in earlier years. This slowdown accounts for the extra pounds. Also, there is a definite metabolic slowdown the older we get, and we need to cut down our calories accordingly. Another factor, but one which I've found to be true quite often, is that people who *have* watched their weight all of their lives on reaching old age tend not to pay quite so much attention to this aspect of their appearance. They often feel that—because of all those years of weight-watching—they now deserve the extra desserts or servings of mashed potatoes. This is quite understandable, but nevertheless is destructive thinking. Old age is just the time when people need to watch their weight the most for health reasons.

It is important, then, to find a healthy and nutritional diet for your life. If you are overweight, you need to begin to reduce sensibly. I want to emphasize *sensibly*, for there are many unhealthy fad diets in existence which will do more harm to your body than you can imagine, regardless of how effective they are in weight reducing. The goal is *healthy* weight reduction. You need a nutritional diet which can eventually be turned into a diet for normal living after you have lost the required amount of weight.

To understand what a healthy diet is, you must first understand what the term "balanced diet" means.

CALORIES

Most people think of calories as evils. This is not entirely warranted, because calories are neither good nor bad. They are units of energy. A calorie is not something you put in your mouth; it is not a piece of pie or a soft drink. A calorie is a way by which we measure the energy value contained in a particular food. Thus, we need a certain number of calories to carry out daily activities. More active people need more calories, and older people generally need fewer calories than younger people. But everyone needs some amount of calories, for without them you would not be getting the needed foods. Calories are a good gauge of how much food you are eating.

However, we cannot base our nutritional plan solely on the amount of calories we are consuming. We must also look at the quality of the foods in which we find those calories. Certain foods contain more nutritive elements than other foods. The amount of nutrition you get for every calorie you consume is a very important part of your diet. Foods which are high in the sugar they contain provide less nutrition and an abundance of calories. In plain terms, eating this kind of food means you are not getting what you paid for. You could eat two rich pieces of cake a day, which might not amount to more than a thousand calories, a sensible amount for a reducing diet, and yet you still would not lose weight because the foods you are eating have little or no nutritive value. So, in a reducing diet, the goal is to reduce the number of calories without sacrificing your level of nutrition. Obviously, then, you must scrutinize your calories to be certain you are eating the foods that will bring you the greatest nutritional benefit for their calories.

SOURCES OF CALORIES

There are three main sources of calories: carbohydrates, proteins, and fats. For a balanced diet, you need some of each, yet the amounts may vary. Every schoolchild knows that an overabundance of fats will be a quick way to put on weight, while a preponderance of protein usually means a healthier body. Lately, many fad diets have come out which severely limit or eliminate altogether carbohydrates. This is a very unhealthy life-scheme, for carbohydrates contain essential elements for a healthy body. So, one must find a balanced diet, using all three sources of calories, and limiting (but not eliminating) the sorts of calories which will give you less nutrition.

CARBOHYDRATES

The body takes carbohydrates into the system in the form of grains such as bread, cereal, rice, and pasta; sugar and sweets of any kinds; and many root vegetables like potatoes and beets. Once in the body, these are transformed into glucose, fructose, and galactose. Carbohydrates are used, with fats, to supply the body with fuel for most physical activities. This is why you will feel particularly energetic after you have eaten a candy bar. The fats and carbohydrates therein raise your energy level, provide you with immediate energy. This is not always the wisest source of energy, because it is quickly burned off.

Carbohydrates are also transformed into supplements of protein building blocks. When your intake of carbohydrates is greater than the energy you are expending, carbohydrates are changed into fat.

FATS

Fats are essential to the diet in certain amounts because special fatty acids cannot be manufactured by the body, and this would mean a great deficiency if you did not consume fats at all. Fats are also a major source of energy, and they are needed for digestion. It is recommended that fats fill from twenty-five to thirty-three percent of your daily intake. There are different classes of fats, however, and some of them are healthier than others. *Saturated fats* are generally not recommended as good sources of fat because they are high in cholesterol, which is cited as a cause of stroke and many other adverse physical reactions or diseases. Saturated fats are usually found in solid types of fats, such as butter, yolks of eggs, and beef fat. They are usually derived from animal sources. The other type of fat is *unsaturated fats*, and these include such products as olive oil, peanut oil, and corn oil.

PROTEIN

Proteins provide the essential units for body maintenance. They are oftentimes referred to as "body building blocks." They are the basis for rejuvenating and replacing body tissues, and for the maintenance of the structure of the skin, hair, nails, connective tissue, and many organs as well. As you can see, an adequate supply of protein is essential to a healthy body. Good sources of protein include many types of beans, most dairy products, whole grains, lean meat, fish, and chicken, and nuts. Obviously, it is best when you are reducing to include in your diet the least caloric sources of protein such as fish, eggs, and chicken. The lecithin in egg yolks makes them ideal for assimilating cholesterol.

A FEW WORDS ABOUT WATER

Many people believe that it is possible to "sweat off" pounds. Exercise indeed is essential when you are dieting to aid the process and to tone your muscles, but the concept that you can shed pounds through shedding water is erroneous. Weight lost through perspiration, either in exercise or in steambaths, is put right back on the moment you have a glass of any kind of liquid. It is a simple fact that your body needs water, at least five or six pints of water each day to replace water it loses through breathing, urinating, excreting, and perspiring. Water is the body's tool for carrying off waste materials. It is nearly impossible to drink too much water because excess water is eliminated, yet you can die if you do not drink enough. So do not try to lose weight through abstaining from water, and do not think that a one-pound loss during the course of a steambath is a permanent or a valuable one.

THE FOUR FOOD GROUPS

Now that we have examined what makes up our foods, it is important to look at those foods themselves. There are four basic food groups: milk; meat; vegetables and fruits; breads and cereals. Within the following descriptions of the food groups, I have included serving amounts for each. It is essential that you get foods from each group each day for a healthy, basic, nutritional plan.

The Milk Group. The milk group includes most dairy products, certainly including cheese, ice cream, and ice milk. However, it must be noticed that here is a dramatic demonstration of "getting what you pay for" in terms of nutrition. You need *two or more* cups of milk products daily, yet if you choose two cups of ice cream, you will certainly be consuming a great number of calories for the small nutritional value. Suggestions include:

1 cup of whole milk	160 calories
1 cup of skim milk, nonfat dry milk, or buttermilk	90 calories
1 cup of chocolate milk	190 calories
1 cup of yogurt	150 calories
1 slice (1 oz.) Swiss cheese	105 calories
½ cup of cottage cheese	130 calories

The Meat Group. Obviously, the products in the meat group include all kinds of beef, veal, lamb, pork, poultry, fish, and eggs, not to mention certain types of beans, peas, and nuts. However, you will get more nutritional value for your calories if you center around the animal products. You should have *two or more servings* of the meat group daily. A serving usually means three ounces of cooked meat, without bone or skin. For dieters, it is best to consume only very lean meats; consequently, eating more chicken and fish is a good idea. Suggestions include:

3 oz. fish or shellfish	200 calories
3 oz. poultry	200 calories
3 oz. cooked lean meat	175 calories
Average hamburger, without bun	245 calories
2 eggs	160 calories

You should also add the correct amount of calories for any oil which you cook these products in. That is why broiled, baked, or boiled methods of cooking are the most advantageous.

The Vegetable and Fruit Group. You must have certain types of vegetables and fruits in certain amounts, but the total is *four servings a day*. This includes one citrus fruit or other source of Vitamin C a day; one dark green or yellow vegetable at least every other day; and other vegetables or fruits to make up the other servings.

Fruits which supply Vitamin C are citrus fruits such as oranges and grapefruits; strawberries, cantaloupe, and vegetables such as broccoli and peppers. The green and yellow vegetables that provide the needed Vitamin A include broccoli, carrots, chard, collards, pumpkin, spinach, sweet potatoes, and winter squash. Fruits supplying Vitamin A include apricots and cantaloupe.

One serving would be one-half cup of the vegetable or the fruit. When we eat many raw fruits such as apples, pears, and peaches, they are not served in cups, but in natural portions. In this case, one serving would be the natural unit, *i.e.*, one banana, one apple, etc. Suggestions include:

6 oz. of unsweetened fruit juice	80 calories
1 banana or grapefruit	80 calories
½ cantaloupe	30 calories
1 peach	40 calories
1 pear, apple, or orange	80 calories
1 cup of canned fruit, unsweetened	40 calories
½ cup of potatoes, corn, or lima beans	70 calories
½ cup of beets, carrots, onions, peas or squash	35 calories
½ cup of leafy greens, cooked green vegetables, eggplant, celery, tomatoes, etc.	20 calories

It is a good idea to eat as many fresh fruits and vegetables as possible, for cooking, and particularly overcooking, tends to dissipate valuable vitamins.

The Bread and Cereal Group. The best foods in this group are the whole grain breads and cereals. This is because they provide protein and also act as roughage for your diet. The American diet, generally, is in bad need of roughage. You should have four servings daily of whole grain breads or cereals. The serving size varies greatly with the type of food you are consuming. That is, a serving of bread would be one slice, a serving of dry cereal would be one ounce, while a serving of cooked cereal, cornmeal, macaroni, noodles, or rice would be one-half to three-quarters of a cup. Suggestions include:

1 slice bread	65 calories
½ cup of cooked cereal	60 calories
1 roll	100 calories
1 cup of dry cereal	100 calories
(remember to add more calories if you are adding fruit, milk, or sugar)	
½ cup of cooked pasta	100 calories

Now that you have an idea of the four basic food groups, you can begin to compile a diet to suit your body and your daily activity. If you are a very active person, you can probably reduce on 1,500 calories a day, but most people should begin with a 1,000-calories-a-day diet. Your plan should include three meals a day. Each meal is important, and you should not get in the habit of skipping any of them. When you skip meals you tend to snack, and snacking invariably means too many calories and not enough nutritional value in your food. Your biggest meal of the day advisedly is lunch. When reducing, it is important also to eat a big breakfast, and a moderate-sized dinner, for the calories you take in at dinner oftentimes are not worked off. One of the unhealthiest things you can do is to eat a large dinner and then sit around the house for the rest of the evening and go directly to bed. All these calories invariably turn right to fat.

The following list is a day-by-day, meal-by-meal, plan for the first week of a diet. You can, of course, substitute where availability or preference varies. Remember, this is not an iron-clad regimen; this should be an enjoyable yet sensible way to reduce.

MONDAY

Breakfast   1 serving fruit, such as orange juice
1 poached egg on
1 slice of whole-wheat toast
1 glass of skim milk
tea or coffee

Lunch   1 sandwich made from 2 slices of whole-wheat bread, 1 teaspoon of margarine or mayonnaise, 2 slices of cheese, and slices of tomato and cucumber
1 pear

Dinner   grilled chicken or lean beef
green beans
carrots
cantaloupe

TUESDAY

Breakfast   tomato juice
bran cereal with skim milk
tea or coffee

Lunch   cold slices of turkey on whole-wheat bread with tomato slices and some sort of spread (margarine, mayonnaise)
carrot sticks
apple

Dinner   barbecued chicken
baked potato
mushrooms and broccoli sautéed
sliced peaches
skim milk

WEDNESDAY

Breakfast   one-half grapefruit
cooked oatmeal with skim milk
coffee or tea

Lunch   cottage cheese and tomato slices
pumpernickel bread
pear

Dinner   veal
rice pilaf
tossed salad of lettuce and tomatoes with oil and
vinegar dressing
sliced nectarines with yogurt

THURSDAY
Breakfast   orange juice
soft-boiled egg
whole-wheat toast
glass of skim milk
tea or coffee
Lunch   grilled cheese sandwich on whole-wheat bread
cole slaw
orange
Dinner   roast turkey
summer squash
wild rice
diet Jell-O

FRIDAY
Breakfast   grapefruit juice
hot, whole-grain cereal
strawberries and milk
coffee or tea
Lunch   vegetable soup
whole-wheat crackers
nuts
pear
Dinner   broiled halibut filets
steamed broccoli with lemon
grilled mushrooms
slices of apple and Cheddar cheese
tea or coffee

SATURDAY
Breakfast   vegetable juice
dry cereal with skim milk
coffee or tea

Lunch   cold slices of chicken in a salad with cucumbers,
               tomatoes, cottage cheese, and a sliced hard-boiled
               egg
               some type of berries
Dinner   broiled lamb chops
               carrots
               green beans
               skim milk
               fresh strawberries and yogurt

SUNDAY
Breakfast cantaloupe
               slices of cheese
               whole-wheat toast
               tea or coffee
Lunch   2-egg omelet made in Teflon pan (without oil or
               butter)
               tomato slices
               glass of skim milk
               apple
               tea or coffee
Dinner   roast chicken
               sliced, cooked carrots
               spinach and mushroom salad
               orange
               tea or coffee

CHAPTER TEN

PHYSICAL AIDS

Even with your newly-acquired mobility and your healthier way of life, you may from time to time undergo periods of extreme pain and inflammation. This is natural, for ultimately we cannot cure arthritis. It is a chronic disease, and consequently the most we can do is to relieve the symptoms. Even with the exercise program, occasional bad periods are unavoidable. It is the nature of the disease.

During these painful periods it is best to refrain from exercising too strenuously. Some gentle movement each day is advisable, but continuation of the program at this time will only irritate the already inflamed joints. Also, it is good to receive at least two hours per day *more rest* than your normal quota of daytime rest. These hours should be spaced out— for example, one in the morning and one in the late afternoon. If you choose to partake of more rest than that, the periods should be spaced out accordingly.

Another kind of aid which you may rely on in these periods is the entire range of physical supports, of which hundreds of types are readily available. I am confident if you have a particular difficulty with basic, functional, everyday life, that a mechanism for the disabled exists to help you. You can find most of this equipment at any hospital or surgical supply store. Usually your physical therapist or your doctor will know of a good outlet in your area. If you discuss your everyday problems with your doctor, he will quite often be able to suggest a particular gadget to aid you.

Again, there exists an entire range, from the basic canes and crutches to more complicated tools. I would like to stress, however, that for the most part these are only temporary measures and physical aids. Although they can become quite useful to you permanently, it is most important not to let this happen. For when you are dependent on an artificial aid, you decrease the range of motion of your limbs and joints, thus decreasing your mobility. This increases your pain and stiffness.

Naturally, there are some aids which some of you who are afflicted with osteoarthritis in its more advanced stages will not be able to do without, and all the better for them, in that case. It is obvious that the use of these special aids for some people represents a very important part of their lives; without them they would be dependent on other people for help in performing the very basic chores of daily life. In these cases we should never underestimate their value, for they become a very important symbol of freedom. They are, in these cases, no more "crutches" than glasses are "crutches" to most of us. Yet I advise those of you who can learn to live without these, except as temporary measures, to do so, even though it may be a little difficult at first.

Perhaps the aid which is most common and the easiest available to you is the cane. The use of a cane can take the weight off a particularly painful joint. There is a wide variety of simple canes which can aid the individual in walking during these very painful periods. Some have hook-type grips, while others are merely knobbed. Also, because it was at one time fashionable to sport a cane, there remain hundreds of types of aesthetically pleasing canes, at various prices and of a wide range of materials. I would advise you, though, to purchase one which is rubber-tipped. The rubber encasement of the lower end helps avoid slipping and skidding, and it is essential in avoiding accidents.

Another more advanced type of cane which has had immense success is the "quad cane." This is a cane with a handle at the top; instead of one prong at the bottom, there are four, each of them spaced to receive an equal amount of the weight, and each, of course, rubber-tipped. The quad cane provides more balance and supports more weight than other types of canes.

If you are more severely afflicted, you may want to investigate the use of crutches. These, too, come in many sizes, altered for many purposes, and made of many materials. Special crutches for sufferers of arthritis are made, usually of aluminum. Also available are crutches into which the individual may slip his arms, if the arms are also afflicted, thus allowing more support from different areas of the body.

In quite severe cases of arthritis, usually those involving hip deformity, a walker may be prescribed. These are frames, usually of sturdy aluminum, upon which the individual puts the full weight of his body through his arms, while taking a step at a time. Once planted, the individual moves the walker one step farther, and continues his progress. Movement by necessity is slow, but it is self-movement, and when leg pain is quite great, this aid is invaluable for the individual's independence.

Another useful temporary aid is the splint. When a joint is undergoing a particularly inflamed or painful period, as I mentioned earlier, an important part of the treatment is extra rest. Often the joints become especially swollen, and to ensure that they remain still, it is important to immobilize them by use of a splint. Splints are worn sporadically during the course of the day, and they can be quite effective at preventing permanent deformity and maintaining mobility of knees, wrists, and fingers.

It is a common misconception that splints are a last resort, and that use of them brings about deformity. The popular opinion seems to be that once you are "locked" in a splint, you must use it constantly and permanently, becoming much like the Man in the Iron Mask. Nothing could be further from the truth. To wear a splint in no way increases the chance of a joint's becoming locked in one position. Actually, it does just the opposite, for it keeps a temporarily inflamed joint immobile, thus preventing overuse. This decreases inflammation, which is the best way to insure that a joint does not become permanently deformed. Extreme inflammation can cause this type of deformity, and so we want to minimize the inflammation by immobilizing the joint. It is a misconception that one should keep one's joints quite active during these bad periods. Rest in splints causes a *decrease* in inflammation and pain, and an *increase* in mobility and function.

Splints are made of several materials, including aluminum, Castex, Lucite, and the more common plaster of paris. A cast is taken of the joint and subsequently a mold is made, making sure the joint is in the proper position for optimum rest. The joint is then periodically enclosed in the splint in a position of normal rest, and counter to that of deformity.

The splint is usually removed several times each day, while the joint is moved in some gentle exercise to maintain range of motion and to prevent rigidity. The amount of movement possible will vary with the amount of tolerance of the patient. The splint is reapplied after the exercise period. The object of this procedure is to maintain mobility in the joint while still providing proper rest for healing.

For less serious instances of inflammation, a lightweight plaster of paris splint can be obtained from a hospital supply store at an inexpensive price. For more specific requirements, an individual mold will be taken of the patient's limb. The splint is made and dried. Once it is ready it is cut into two halves, called bivalving it, and in this way it can easily be taken on and off of the joint at any time during the day or night.

Splinting should be prescribed and supervised by a doctor, because there is a particular method of treatment involved. He will decide at what angle your limb should be maintained, and for how long. Generally, new splints are cast approximately once a week in order to maintain the progress which has been achieved, instead of continuing to employ the same splints with less desirable angles of flexion.

Usually a splint can only be employed on smaller joints, including wrist, finger, knee, and ankle joints. Obviously, it is impractical to think of splinting a larger joint such as the hip joint, or the spine.

If the knee joint is terribly inflamed, extra difficulty may occur. If, after the pain and swelling go down, a certain amount of deformity has set in, the individual may have specific problems with walking. At this point and until the patient has regained full use of his legs, the doctor may prescribe a durable and strong splint to be worn during the day. Often these splints are made from plastic. They lend much support to a knee joint during the walking process. In this way, the patient is able to walk without undergoing severe strain, until the muscles surrounding the afflicted area have recovered enough to be able to support the joint in a normal fashion.

Also along the lines of casting splints is a new process by which people with deformed feet may find shoes to fit them. As many of you know only too well, when arthritis strikes the feet and toe joints, it not only provides much pain and distress, but it also makes it quite difficult to buy shoes which fit or which are comfortable. And well-fitting shoes are essential to a person's mobility, particularly if that person's feet hurt already from arthritis.

Until recently there were few solutions to this problem. It is impossible for people who have arthritic or other deformities of the feet to find suitable shoes in ordinary stores. And we all are aware of how expensive it is for an individual to have shoes made expressly for him. However, there is now a solution to this problem. There has been developed a process of taking casts of the feet from plaster of paris. After the impressions are made, they are then sent to a shoe factory, where shoes are manufactured for these particular feet. This method is nowhere near as expensive as having a private shoemaker tailor the shoes just for your feet and make them by hand.

Apart from these therapeutic devices, there is also a wealth of tools which have been manufactured to make your home situation more comfortable. There is such a wide range that it would be impossible to list them all here. A much wiser solution would be for you to ask your doctor or physical therapist to recommend an occupational therapist for you. You might also call the arthritis or orthopedic clinic at your local hospital for a recommendation.

Occupational therapists are trained in reviving the day-to-day abilities of the patient. They teach the disabled how to cope with any level of disability, so as to render them as independent as possible. This includes anything from teaching a person to button his clothes to teaching the use of the right or left hand as a replacement for the lost capacity of the major hand, to teaching people to get in and out of bath-tubs. Consequently, these people have at their fingertips information regarding the many tools for home use. An occupational therapist will gladly come for a home visit, simply to chat with the arthritic to discover what the major home-living difficulties are and to give suggestions for their improvement. It is particularly helpful for the occupational therapist to come to the home, in order to better examine the living situation and determine what modifications can be made. He or she will then make many useful suggestions.

Several simple alterations can make all the difference in a

comfortable home life. The kitchen is a major source of problems for many people who are afflicted with arthritis. It is often poorly organized, which may make little difference for the unafflicted housewife, but for someone who needs to take as few steps as possible, every poorly-arranged cupboard is an extra burden.

Often women arrange their kitchens according to tradition, in the manner their mothers arranged their own kitchens, rather than according to function. For example, the bread container will be at one end of the kitchen, while the toaster and the spreads for bread are at the other. This may seem trivial, but correcting this arrangement could save the individual many painful, unnecessary steps. In all, the extra walking involved may amount to *miles* each day, carrying pots from stove to sink and back, and carrying food from the refrigerator across the kitchen to the work space. All that is required to correct this is rearrangement of the kitchen. This may take an afternoon to accomplish, but it will be well worth the effort in saved motions.

For the rearrangement, make sure you have a work space next to your stove and sink. An optimal condition would be to have the space between these two appliances, and, large enough to hold two cooking processes at once. This will enable you to move things across surfaces to their destinations, rather than forcing you to lift and carry heavy objects. Also, remember to place your small appliances near the cupboards which contain the main ingredients to be cooked or mixed in those appliances. For example, if you make a morning milk, honey, and wheatgerm drink in your blender, don't put the blender in a niche away from the refrigerator. Other simple considerations of this type can eliminate wasted, and often painful, motions.

Many special cooking utensils have been created for people with arthritic problems. For example, there are knives, spoons, and spatulas with quite thick handles, so people who normally could not close their fingers around the handles can do so. Special spoons and other flatware whose handles are at a different angle from the usual one are also available. Of course, many lightweight pots and pans exist for people who cannot easily move the very heavy ones.

The bathroom is another room where arthritics have a great deal of difficulty. Often it is embarrassing for the individual to discuss this, even with members of the immediate family. That is why I have suggested a meeting with an occupational therapist, for he or she deals in these problems every day. Solving them is what the job entails. Never feel sheepish about discussing such a problem with your occupational therapist.

Individuals with severe hip or knee pain may have problems in getting on and off the toilet. There are several modifications which can be inexpensively and easily installed in your bathroom to aid you. A rail, generally about ten to twelve inches in length, can be put on the wall for you to grab for support in lifting yourself on and off the seat. Another device is the raised toilet seat, which is held by a frame of metal or plastic five or six inches above the normal seat. It fits conveniently over a normal toilet seat, and can be removed by simply lifting it up.

A more serious problem is that in many homes with second stories the bathroom becomes inaccessible because it is on the second floor, and the arthritic cannot mount the stairs. This problem is not insurmountable either. Many inexpensive and completely hygienic chemical, portable toilets are now on the market. They can be moved to the patient and, after use, placed somewhere inconspicuous, all without any unpleasantness or difficulty.

Also, a person who is severely crippled in his shoulders or back may find after-bathroom hygiene a problem. This is a common occurrence, and many forms of *bidets* are manufactured which solve this problem. They come equipped with a special spray of water, which is followed by gentle, warm air for drying.

Also available are various constructions of bath seats and rails. The rails enable the person to help himself into the tub. The seats are for people who are in more pain and cannot bend their joints far enough to get down into the tub. The seat fits conveniently and easily across the tub so that the person can sit on top of it, yet still be in close proximity to the water. These are constructed both of metal and of sturdy, durable plastic. They are usually white, though special colors can be obtained, and are aesthetically pleasing. Many people who are not afflicted with arthritis prefer to bathe in this fashion.

Doorknobs often pose a large problem for people with arthritis of the hands and wrists. Many times it is simply too difficult to make the required twisting motion. Consequently lever-type handles can be installed in place of knobs. These require merely a slight downward motion to activate them.

The range of home devices is unbelievable. There exist special handles for turning problem faucets, devices for removing stockings and for putting them on, devices for opening low oven doors, and of course, a variety of cosmetic devices for personal hygiene. Many times an individual will not be able to use a hair brush or comb, or a toothbrush. There are all manner of utensils with special handles for accomplishing these tasks.

Recreational activities have not been ignored either. For instance, many avid card players find to their disappointment that they can no longer hold cards during a game of bridge. A simple card-holding device has been developed for this purpose. It is in the form of a block of wood with slits or metal prongs into which any number of cards may fit. These are finely made and unobtrusive gadgets.

Elastic or support stockings represent another medical aid. These can be quite effective in preventing or relieving varicose veins, and in lending much support to muscles that are just regaining strength. If you have to be on your feet much of the day, or if you have a good bit of walking to do, wearing these stockings can give lots of relief to legs, and more important, to joints that would otherwise be exhausted and painful by the end of the day. The only disadvantage in these stockings is that if you wear a pair that are too tight, they will cut the circulation off in your legs. This reverses their effectiveness, rendering them destructive. With decreased blood flow your muscles cannot regain their strength, nor can your joints maintain any kind of mobility. So it is very important to choose scrupulously a stocking that is neither too tight nor too loose.

As regards all of these physical aids, I would like to reiterate that they do have particular advantages, and for some people they may be essential. It is, of course, better to use one of these aids and still be independently mobile than to depend on other people for help, for this latter form of dependence tends to undermine self-esteem. However, it is equally essential that those of you who do not absolutely need these aids, *not* use them permanently, for *to become needlessly dependent on any of them counteracts their purpose, and can be self-defeating*.

CHAPTER ELEVEN

YOUR OUTLOOK FOR AN ACTIVE FUTURE

I wish I could demonstrate for you in a more dramatic way the effectiveness of the exercise program described in this book. I would like to be able to give you a one hundred percent sales pitch like so many advertisers do every time they come up with a new scheme for your health. But that would be more "selling" than hard facts, and I am sure that you have had your share of the hard sell as concerns your arthritis. What you need now is the simple truth. I cannot "sell" the exercise program any more than to explain it, and to assure you that if you follow it consistently, you *will* achieve results. I have seen this happen with so many of my friends. They would go for years trying all manner of drugs and fad treatments which promised to relieve their pains and sometimes even to cure the disease. When this failed, they ended up merely learning to live with the disease, not even thinking to try the simplest, most healthy method of treatment—*proper exercise.*

This, unfortunately, is often the way in life. We try all the complicated solutions before we ever get around to thinking about the simplest and most effective ones. Exercise has always been a health-builder for the human body. The ancient Greeks well understood the importance of a healthy body as well as a healthy, well-developed mind. This is of course still true. Our bodies need a certain amount of exercise to maintain themselves simply so we can get from place to place during our daily activities. All too often in our society we ignore this fact and let our daily quota of active exercise diminish until it is nearly non-existent.

The stiffness of arthritis many times exists simply from years of non-use of those afflicted joints, and the pain often comes simply from an excess amount of weight being carried by those joints. That is why you need exercise to relieve that stiffness and the pain.

Osteoarthritis, as we have seen, is a degeneration of the joints in the body, caused because the lubricating fluids cease to function as they should. To this day no cure has been found for this disease, but neither is it a fatal one—you cannot die from osteoarthritis. These are the simple facts, and if anyone tries to convince you that a particular drug or practice will *cure* you of osteoarthritis, you can be sure he is a charlatan.

However grim this fact may sound, it still remains that the *symptoms* of arthritis can be assuaged, which, for all intents and purposes, is a cure of a kind. You can, through the daily practice of a series of mild and easy exercises, gain new, wider ranges of motion in all of your joints, and with this agility eliminate the pain.

This sensible exercise plan, with temporary adjuncts of heat treatments and a permanent proper plan of nutrition, can develop for you a normal, healthy, and happy life.

I would like to emphasize that these exercises are not difficult. They are not strenuous. They will not hurt. You have absolutely nothing to lose by starting your program of exercise *today*, this afternoon. Set aside fifteen minutes and begin to choose, and to experiment with, the exercises prescribed for your particular condition. You may say that you really haven't got the time today, that you will start this weekend. *It is essential that you begin now.* Fifteen minutes is a very short time compared to all the long and frustrating nights that you have lain in bed, not able to sleep nor to move for the pain.

You could begin right this moment. Stand up in the center of the room and start with the "wake-up" exercises. These will take only a couple of moments, and yet I know after you have performed them you will already feel better. Once you have done this you will have begun the program, and most important, you will have taken the initiative to change your life in this easy, but very dramatic way. Good luck!

CHAPTER TWELVE

A CHECKLIST

As we have seen throughout this book, if you suffer from osteoarthritis and want to secure relief from the pain and stiffness, one of the essential things you must do is to change your attitudes toward your lifestyle. You must rearrange your thoughts, and thus your life, so that you curb any sedentary or destructive activity in which you are participating.

The following is a checklist of habits by which you can examine the quality of your daily activities. If you find that you are engaging in too many bad habits and not enough of the good, you should make an effort not just to break these but to begin to live the life of a more active person. I assure you that you will become a healthier, happier individual.

THE CHECKLIST

1. Do you find yourself watching television for more than an hour at a time?

    or

    Do you split up your television-watching time with other activities, such as washing the dishes, taking walks, or simply choosing programs at different times of the day?

2. Do you watch television during that hour without getting up from your seat at all?

or

Do you walk about during commercials, or at least stand or stretch, perhaps doing some of the stretching exercises which I outlined earlier?

3. Do you find yourself saying no when friends invite you for outdoor sports activities, giving the excuse that you are too old or too stiff?

or

Do you accept these dates, and sometimes suggest them yourself, knowing that, in moderation, no such activity is for only the young and agile?

4. Do you simply prefer to be in the house?

or

Do you balance your time between being outdoors and being inside?

5. When you are at home, do you find yourself bored much of the time?

or

When you are bored, or finished with your household activities, do you step outside for fresh air?

6. Do you talk on the phone for hours with your friends who live nearby?

or

Do you go visit them instead?

7. Do you associate relaxation with sitting or lying down?

or

Do you acknowledge the many other forms of healthy exercise which are also relaxing?

8. Do you sleep more than nine hours a night?

or

Do you get just as much sleep as you need and no more, thus avoiding waking up with the morning "drugged" feeling?

9. Do you go out to films and restaurants only?

or

Do you go out during the daytime, particularly on the weekends, and participate in daytime, motion-oriented activities, instead of the sitting-oriented ones?

10. Do you automatically jump into your car or on the bus when there is an errand to be done?

or

If it is within walking distance, do you *walk instead of riding*?

11. Do you sit in your office all day, behind your desk, without getting up for stretches?

or

Do you utilize your time and organize your activities so that you get a variety of movements, as well as trying a few stretching exercises from time to time?

12. Do you get home from work and collapse in a chair until dinnertime and then eat, watch television, and go to bed?

or

Do you get home from work and go out for a healthy, leisurely walk around your neighborhood, coupled perhaps with some conversation with your friends?

13. If you are feeling "lazy" on a particular day, do you lie in bed and wait for the feeling to pass?

or

Do you get out of bed and begin some mild, wake-up exercises to get the energy flow in your body going, so you will not waste the entire day?

THE ARTHRITIS FOUNDATION

While the self-help program I have outlined in this book is an invaluable tool when properly used, your local chapter of the Arthritis Foundation can be of great assistance to you in finding the necessary medical care to go with my program, and the Foundation offers a wide range of services to those afflicted with arthritis. Some chapters have even organized clubs, where people with the shared problem of arthritis to face can get together and help each other. To find out if there is a chapter in your community, consult your telephone directory or write to the national headquarters (The Arthritis Foundation, Inc., 3400 Peachtree Road, N.E., Atlanta, Georgia 30326) for the location of the chapter nearest you. The Foundation also supplies patients with leaflets, reprints and other literature on arthritis.

Index